CLINICAL MEDICAL ETHICS

Exploration and Assessment

Edited by

Terrence F. Ackerman
Glenn C. Graber
Charles H. Reynolds
David C. Thomasma

THE UNIVERSITY OF TENNESSEE
Inter-Campus Graduate Program in Medical Ethics

UNIVERSITY
PRESS OF
AMERICA

LANHAM • NEW YORK • LONDON

British Cataloging in Publication Information Available

Co-published by arrangement with
The University of Tennessee
Inter-Campus Graduate Program in Medical Ethics

Library of Congress Cataloging in Publication Data

Clinical medical ethics.

Includes index.
1. Medical ethics—Congresses.   2. Medicine, Clinical
—Moral and ethical aspects—Congresses.   I. Ackerman,
Terrence F., 1949-   .   II. University of Tennessee,
Knoxville. Inter-Campus Graduate Program in Medical
Ethics.   [DNLM: 1. Ethics, Medical.   W   50   C6414]
R724.C526   1987   174'.2   86-28176
ISBN 0-8191-6039-3 (alk. paper)
ISBN 0-8191-6040-7 (pbk. : alk. paper)

TABLE OF CONTENTS

An increasing number of medical ethicists are becoming involved in the clinical setting. Their involvement in clinical care and health professional education raises a number of important issues about the objectives of clinical ethics teaching, the role responsibilities of ethica consultants, and the usefulness of moral theory in clinical problem solving. The essays in this volume assess the present state of clinical teaching, consultation, and research activities in medical ethics and explore the issues such activities raise.

This collection of essays grew out of a conference held in August 1982 under the sponsorship of the University of Tennessee Inter-Campus Graduate Program in Medical Ethics. The conference was structured around three "Exchanges" between professionals knowledgeable in the field of medical ethics, who represent diverse philosophical perspectives and traditions. The topics and speakers for these three sessions, and the guiding questions posed to them were as follows:

EXCHANGE #1

TOPIC: Does a Clinical Role for Medical Ethics Violate or Enhance Therapeutic Relationships?

QUESTIONS: The American Hospital Association's "Patient's Bill of Rights" states: "Those not directly involved in [the patient's] care must have the permission of the patient to be present" at case discussion, consultation, examination and treatment. Could a medical ethics consultant be construed as one who is "directly involved in" care? Alternatively, is the function of the medical ethicist so remote from care that it would be inappropriate even to ask the patient for permission to have him/her present? Is there really a need for medical ethics professionals to be at the bedside? If so, what is the basis of this need? Do the benefits outweigh the costs in terms of invasion of patient privacy and intrusion into the physician-patient relationship?

SPEAKERS: John A. Robertson and Robert M. Veatch

EXCHANGE #2

TOPIC: Teaching Medical Ethics in the Clinical Setting: Objectives, Strategies, Qualifications

QUESTIONS: Can persons without medical training understand enough about cases to address the ethical issues
helpfully, or will they be hopelessly dependent on
clinicians to highlight the ethical issues for them (in
which case, a vital step in ethical analysis will have
already been completed)? Which is the soundest
approach to training medical ethics teachers and
researchers for the future -- should we begin with
ethicists and seek to train them in the rudiments of
medical science, or should we attempt instead to
recruit physicians to study ethics? What are the
advantages and limitations of team teaching in this
field? What is the ideal combination of ethical theory
and case studies in medical ethics teaching at various
levels?

SPEAKERS: Howard Brody and Arthur Caplan

EXCHANGE #3

TOPIC: Theory/Practice Dialectic in Clinical Medical
Ethics: The Case Format

QUESTIONS: Is the case focus of most current medical
ethics discussion **philosophically** respectable?
Casuistry has traditionally been thought to be among
the least interesting enterprises in philosophical
ethics. Is this true of the use of cases in medical
ethics, or (as some argue) is the case focus the
strength of the field--offering the potential of creative new approaches to ethics that move beyond the
bounds of traditional theory?

SPEAKERS: Kai Nielsen and Albert Jonsen

Most of the remainder of the conference was devoted to
small-group working sessions in which issues raised in the
Exchanges, and other issues within the scope of the conference
topics, were addressed from the perspective of each participant's
professional activities. It is impossible to communicate the
lively discussions that took place in these working sessions
among subgroups of the 175 professionals who attended the conference, but the essays contributed by the four editors incorporate elements of these discussions, as well as reflections on
the exchanges, independent thinkers on these topics, and information about elements of the University of Tennessee Inter-Campus
Graduate Program in Medical Ethics.

ACKNOWLEDGEMENTS: The editors are grateful to the Rockefeller Foundation for financial support for the conference and this publication (Grant No. GA HUM 8133). Planning for the conference and research on the editors' essays was supported by Program Implementation Grant (#ED-*0652-78) from the National Endowment for the Humanities. The UTK Department of Conferences contributed greatly to the smooth working of the conference. Assistance with conference planning and direction of small-group working sessions was provided by our colleagues and graduate students in the UT Inter-Campus Gradute Program in Medical Ethics, especially: Alfred D. Beasley, J. Thompson Brown, John W. Davis, John A. Eaddy, Rem B. Edwards, H. Phillips Hamlin, Richard Sherlock, and Carson Strong. We also want to thank Mrs. Dolores Scates for her expert secretarial assistance in preparing this volume for publication.

We owe a special debt of gratitude to Dr. John W. Prados, Vice President for Academic Affairs and Research of the University of Tennessee. His encouragement and support at every stage have been vital to our success in developing and maintaining a complex multi-campus, interdisciplinary program of study and research within this institution. Dr. Prados represents administration at its finest: a deep personal commitment to educational ideas in general and to the integration of humanities into professional education in particular, an engaging and supportive style of interaction, an eagerness to facilitate faculty initiatives in every way feasible, a straight account of the limits of feasibility.

In recognition of this support of our program activities, we gratefully dedicate this volume to him.

TEACHING MEDICAL ETHICS IN THE CLINICAL SETTING
OBJECTIVES, STRATEGIES, QUALIFICATIONS

Glenn C. Graber

Two elements in the title of this section serve to limit the focus of our attention here. First, we are dealing with **teaching** medical ethics. Thus, we need not concern ourselves directly with scholarly activities in medical ethics. Nor need we consider in itself the role scholars in medical ethics are occasionally called on to fill as consultants on particular clinical cases.[1] We are also not directly concerned with the contribution of medical ethics to the formulation of public policy.[2] Of course, each of these and other initiallyexcluded elements may turn out to have relevance to the task of teaching; and, insofar as this is the case, they do come within our purview. (We shall consider the relevance for teaching of these elements in part B of the present essay).

Second, we are here dealing with teaching medical ethics **in the clinical setting** -- not in the lecture hall or the seminar room. This emphasis, in turn, serves to delimit our focus in two ways. (a) It suggests that the constituency to be taught is practicing or in-training health care professionals, rather than a general audience of students with a variety of points of interest in and points of view towards the issues of biomedical ethics. (b) The exigencies of clinical training and practice influence the methods and strategies to be employed in teaching. Here again, other teaching settings and strategies may be brought into the discussion whenever they become relevant to our primary concern; but they will not be the central focus of these remarks.*

---

*The University of Tennessee program of graduate studies in philosophy with concentration in medical ethics, which enrolls chiefly students with a background in humanities disciplines, also involves considerable clinical teaching. Thus it might be appropriate to include discussion of this as well. However, the nature of this teaching is markedly different from that oriented towards clinical practitioners. Furthermore, its goal is to prepare these students to engage in clinical teaching of practitioners. Therefore, I shall postpone discussion of these teaching activities until part C of the essay, when we discuss qualifications for clinical medical ethics teaching.

A. OBJECTIVES OF CLINICAL MEDICAL ETHICS TEACHING

The students to be taught, then, are those training to become clinical health care practitioners. To date, teaching efforts in bioethics have been directed almost exclusively towards two fields of clinical practice -- medicine and nursing. However, faculty in the UT program have also been involved with a number of other clinical fields, including dentistry, pharmacy, medical social work, chaplaincy, physical therapy, laboratory technology, and other "allied" health professions. Similar objectives and strategies apply to all these fields, so I shall include them all in this discussion.

The overall objective of health professions training programs is to develop the skills necessary to enable graduates to provide quality patient care, health education and planning, and research. As a component of the training program, medical ethics teaching must take as its primary goal the aim of making its distinctive contribution to this overall objective.

I would anticipate three sorts of objections that might arise to the choice of this -- fairly pragmatic -- overall goal. First, some will question whether philosophy has anything distinctive to contribute to the skills of clinical decision-making and practice.[3] Second, some will charge that it represents a prostitution of philosophy to put it to the service of such practical goals. Philosophy ought to be taught and studied **for its own sake**, it is argued, or for such lofty purposes as to satisfy one's deepest yearnings of curiosity or to enrich and extend one's understanding of the world. The third objection is closely related to the second. To bring the hallowed traditions of philosophy into the service of a technical training program, it is charged, runs the danger of reducing them to a series of "techniques" -- thereby leaving out the fundamental background ruminations which form the heart and soul of the philosophical enterprise.[4] Rather than pausing here to address these objections, I shall offer remarks about them at relevant points throughout the discussion and summarize my replies at the end of section B of the essay.[5]

The first step in further defining this overall goal is to notice the pervasiveness of value judgments and ethical principles in clinical decisions and practices. I would contend (perhaps thereby disagreeing with my colleague Terrence Ackerman in his essay elsewhere in this volume and in certain other of his writings)[6] that **every** clinical decision--even those which are unproblematic -- has significant value and ethical components. In this, I agree with Edmund D. Pellegrino and David C. Thomasma when they say:

2

> Medicine is intrinsically a moral activity
> because all its many functions converge upon
> one end: making a decision for a particular
> person who presents himself in need, as a
> **patient**, someone bearing distress or
> disease. Everything the physician does, all
> his skill and knowledge, must focus on a
> choice of which of the many possible actions
> should be taken for this patient. What is
> the right decision, the one which is good for
> this patient -- not patients in general, not
> what is good for the physician, for the
> science of medicine, or even for society as a
> whole.[7]

Eric Cassell makes a similar point: "I believe that medicine is inherently a moral profession -- or a moral-technical profession, if you wish...because it has directly to do with the welfare and the good of others."[8] Cassell adds elsewhere in the same volume:

> Perhaps that would not be so if in each case
> there was only one right decision or only one
> correct course of action, but in medicine
> there are frequently several possible courses
> of action, each of which is technically cor-
> rect. Or there may be only one technically
> proper decision but several different ways of
> implementing it, each of which would affect
> the life of the patient somewhat
> differently.[9]

Thus, in every clinical encounter, the technical judgments of diagnosis (including second-level judgments about one's degree of assurance in the diagnostic judgment and the decision whether to undertake additional diagnostic procedures to increase the level of confidence), enumeration of alternatives for treatment, prediction of the efficacy and risks of these alternatives and the like are thoroughly woven together with judgments about values and ethical principles (e.g., benefits and harms to the patient and others, implications for the patient's autonomy, privacy, and/or other of his/her rights). Thus one cannot adequately consider the technical dimensions of clinical judgment in isolation from their normative dimensions. Indeed, I would contend that the latter -- normative -- sort of consideration should be the **dominant** concern and should govern judgments of the former, technical sort, since the primary goal of clinical encounters is to maximize the welfare and to preserve or enhance the moral standing of the patient.

3

However, these normative aspects of clinical decisions often escape notice, both in the course of training and in professional practice. They are tacitly assumed to be of a piece with the technical aspects, and they are often subsumed together with them under the label "medical indications and contraindications."[10]

Clearly, these aspects of clinical decisions cannot be adequately analyzed until they are noticed. The first more specific objective, therefore, for teaching medical ethics in the clinical setting is:

(1) To make students (clinical practitioners) aware of the ethical and value dimensions of clinical decisions so they are able (a) to identify which aspects of decisions are technical in nature and which are ethical and (b) to explain how the technical aspects and the ethical aspects are related to each other.[11]

Once this dimension of clinical decisions has been brought to attention, then the normative elements can be dealt with. It is to this end that I direct the second more specific objective of clinical medical ethics teaching:

(2) To develop skills in analyzing and bringing to a sound and generally satisfactory resolution the value and ethical aspects of clinical decisions, in a way corresponding to the way clinical practitioners are taught to handle the technical aspects.

The desired outcome, then, is sound clinical decisions and practice. The distinctive contribution of medical ethics is to focus upon the value and ethical dimensions of these decisions. How this is to be accomplished can be spelled out in a series of even more specific objectives. (I will describe this even further in part B of this essay, when I turn to strategies and methods of clinical teaching).

The first such objective I would stress is:

(2a) To develop awareness of personal values and principles.

One significant barrier to explicit and cogent analysis of the ethical and value dimensions of clinical decisions is the fact that personal values and principles (including some which have been acquired in the process of professional socialization) may lie "submerged" in one's thinking and thereby may influence

4

decisions unnoticed. One important step toward overcoming this situation is to make the practitioner aware of his/her personal values and principles and the way in which these influence the decisions s/he makes.

But awareness by itself is not enough. One must also **deal with** these elements, which leads us to a second objective:

(2b) **To develop skills in critically examining personal values and principles.**

The goal here is not so much to **change** the student's pattern of values and beliefs (although some alteration of content may be nearly inevitable in the process), as it is to lead the student to explore the fundamental "way of life"[12] which underlies his/her normative perspective.

One chief way of accomplishing this, and at the same time another important step towards achieving the larger objective is:

(2c) **To become aware of alternative points of view on value questions, and to probe their implications for concrete health care decisions.**

One of the most effective ways of bringing one's personal values and principles into awareness is by comparing and contrasting one's own patterns of thinking and initial conclusions with various alternative systems of normative thought. At the same time, exposure to systems that differ from one's own offers options for making changes in one's own beliefs.

Exposure to details of alternative normative systems of thought -- and especially the exercise of probing their application to concrete health care decisions -- provides the opportunity for something approximating John Rawls's method of "reflective equilibrium"[13] to come into play. One is led to strive to construct a system of normative thinking which is both consistent in itself and fits in with the conclusions one is inclined to draw in concrete cases.

However, focus on conclusions alone is insufficient. The reasoning behind a conclusion must also be noticed and analyzed. This leads us to the next more specific objective:

(2d) **To detect common errors of reasoning and common patterns of reasoning in discussions of ethical and value issues.**

I have in mind here, not only issues in meta-ethics (which may or may not necessarily arise in a central way), but also points about the "logic" of rights claims, the structure, workings, and implications of utility-balancing procedures, and the like.

Another skill necessary in moral analysis is conceptual analysis, which is the subject of the next specific objective:

(2e) To develop awareness of, and skill in analyzing, distinctive concepts which arise in
normative thinking.

An understanding of general concepts like "rights," "autonomy," "responsibility," and the like -- along with insights into the way in which analyses of these notions will embody a normative perspective -- is an important component of careful normative thinking. Further, analysis of concepts like "death," "health," and "professional" are essential to unravel certain key clinical medical ethics issues.

These sub-objectives must, further, all be brought together and made to bear on the concrete clinical decision -- which brings us to the last of these more specific objectives:

(2f) To develop skills of analyzing ethical
issues, as they arise in particular clinical
cases.

Finally, I would add one more general objective:

(3) To develop skills of communicating the
results of these analyses:

(3a) to patients and families.
(3b) to fellow-practitioners.
(3c) to the general public.

These communications skills are of central importance in clinical practice. Given the legal and ethical requirements of informed consent, it is not enough for a practitioner to satisfy his/her own mind about the correctness of a treatment decision. The patient must agree, as well -- and perhaps also the patient's family and close friends. Thus the practitioner must be able to communicate both the results of his/her decision and the rea-soning behind it in order to adequately inform the patient and enlist his/her consent [Objective 3a]. As Pellegrino and Thomasma point out:

> Once the ethical and logical possibility and "strength" of arguments for one action over another are assessed by dialectic, then the reasoning becomes "rhetorical" -- in the sense of artful persuasion, or relating a dialectically established decision to prudent action, generating belief of another kind from scientific or logical cogency, belief that this particular action should be taken in preference to all others.[14]

Further, given the co-operative nature of today's clinical practice -- with a wide variety of professionals (each with his/her own specific domain of expertise, skill, and consequent responsibility) involved in the care of each patient -- communication between practitioners [Objective 3b] is becoming increasingly important even when each is conceived as operating independently within his/her own domain. And the emerging implementation of a team approach to clinical decision-making and practice makes intra-professional communication even more vital. If a group is attempting to make a decision jointly, each member must be able to state and defend his/her view on the issue to the others.

Finally, the growing public interest in and discussion of normative issues in clinical health care gives rise to a necessity for practitioners to explain and defend their positions on these issues to a general audience [Objective 3c].

B. STRATEGIES FOR CLINICAL MEDICAL ETHICS TEACHING

These objectives, in turn, help define the methods and strategies to be employed in clinical ethics teaching. To begin with one negative example: the goal is not to turn practitioners-in-training into philosophers, and thus there is no intrinsic necessity to expose students to the great classics of Western philosophy. No matter how enriching, intriguing, or mind-expanding these classics might be in their own right, they have no place in clinical teaching except insofar as they serve the objectives enumerated above. (This way of thinking can be extremely valuable to us as teachers -- compelling us to re-evaluate the classics we so dearly love from the perspective of their applicability to clinical ethics issues. I am convinced that the true classics will pass this test, and thus will find a place in applied ethics teaching -- although the method of their presentation will have to be changed from the traditional focus on these writings as items of intrinsic interest to one which highlights their application to concrete issues).

There most certainly is a place within clinical ethics teaching for examination of ethical theories in some depth. The goals of making students aware of alternative points of view on value questions [Objective 2c] and of acquainting them with patterns of ethical reasoning [Objective 2d] would be inadequately met if students never were exposed to a variety of the classical ethics theories of Western culture, such as those of Aristotle, Kant, and Mill. Without some considerable awareness of these systems of thought, we could not say that students had received full and rich exposure to alternative points of view and patterns of reasoning.

One deficiency I find in much of the existing medical ethics literature is its superficiality with regard to points of ethical theory. Too often, concrete cases are addressed in terms of a narrow understanding of middle-level principles such as autonomy or veracity, without any effort to probe the deeper meaning of these principles by examining their roots in an ethical theory such as that of Kant. Or, what amounts to the same error, a mechanical and highly selective utilitarian calculation is offered without probing the full implications for the issue of the root notions within classical utilitarianism. Textbooks in medical ethics often contain reference to some fundaments of these ethical theories (usually in the introductory chapter), but connections are not usually established between these points and discussions of concrete ethical issues in the body of the book.

The only questions which arise about this matter concern (1) when and (2) in what form these theories should be presented. I shall discuss the latter first.

(2) It would, of course be ideal in many ways to have students read such classics as Nichomachean Ethics, the Foundations of the Metaphysics of Morals, and Utilitarianism (and we might take it as an indication of success in our teaching if some students are prompted to tackle these books on their own initiative), but I am not convinced that grappling with the problems of appropriation and interpretation of these texts is either essential to an understanding of the points of view represented in them or a wise pedagogical strategy for clinical ethics teaching. It can suffice to present summaries and/or schematic sketches of the ethical theories embodied in these texts -- perhaps accompanied by brief selections from the originals to give some of their "flavor" and substance.

This approach invites critical reaction from one's peers, since any summary of a subtle and complex ethical theory is bound to run roughshod over many points of scholarly controversy. It

8

is probably healthy to make students aware of **some** of these controversies of interpretation, since this can further extend their understanding of the variety of points of view that are possible on normative issues; but I am convinced that it would be a serious mistake to import narrow issues of scholarly debate into the context of clinical medical ethics teaching.[15] The primary emphasis, instead, ought to be on gaining sufficient understanding of the ethical theories studied to be able to see their implications for and applications to concrete clinical decisions.

(1) The question of **when** to teach this material is a complicated one to answer. Let me first make several comments relevant to this question, and then I will offer a proposal in some detail. (a) I am convinced that it would be a mistake to offer a heavy dose of ethical theory at the initiation of clinical ethics teaching. Without first being convinced of its relevance to clinical decisions, students are unlikely to be motivated to grapple with such abstract and abstruse material. The temptation to begin with theory stems, I think, from two sources: first, the sense that this is foundational and needs to be available to draw upon in discussing concrete issues in clinical ethics; and second, the fact that this is the medical ethics teacher's "home turf" -- the component of the material that s/he is most familiar and comfortable with as a result of his/her professional training. However, both of these sources of temptation should be resisted. It is far more important to create an appetite for this material in the student before introducing it -- even if this means that discussion of some concrete issues have to be allowed to proceed without benefit of useful background concepts and principles -- rather than to permit niceties of logical priority to rule. Further, it is also pedagogically more sound to begin the discussion on the **student's** "home turf" (i.e., the clinical decision in a concrete case) -- even at the cost, on the part of the instructor, of some anxiety and sense of not being fully in control of the material.

(b) We should be cautious about appropriating the model of other components of health professions training. Brody's account, in his essay in this section,[16] of the typical medical student and the typical structure of medical education are painfully accurate. And others of the health professions are all too ready to import the undesirable elements of this model into their training programs in an attempt to mimic medical education. As a partial corrective, Brody recommends that medical ethics teaching be patterned on the models of "the good basic medical science teacher" and/or "the good consultant."

There is much in Brody's suggestion with which I agree wholeheartedly, but I want to enter a caution or two about it as well. Even at its best, the model of the good medical science teacher suggests a division between theory and clinical practice which is unfortunate in any of the disciplines involved -- and especially so in medical ethics. In many health professions training programs, medical ethics is consigned wholly to the basic science years. The chief problems with this, as I see it, are two: First, this puts medical ethics study into direct competition with that mass of other theoretical material which students are expected to master during these years of study. And, since the relevance to clinical practice of the technical material in bio-chemistry, physiology, anatomy, etc. is already widely accepted among students (even when what they are being taught consists of minutiae and esoterica which will, in fact, have little or no utility in clinical practice), medical ethics is likely to receive low priority in such a competition for student's time and attention. Thus, at the very least, medical ethics teachers will have to work strenuously to convince students of the relevance of this area of study to clinical practice.

The second problem with confining medical ethics study to the preclinical, basic science years is that -- like much of the minutiae and esoterica of the basic science courses -- this material will be put out of mind as soon as the courses are completed and grades are duly recorded, and thus it is unlikely to be incorporated into clinical decision-making in the years of clinical study and in later professional practice.

It is essential, then, in order to achieve the objectives set out in Section A above, that preliminary exposure to medical ethics be reinforced and further developed during the clinical training years. Several training programs (including the UT Center for the Health Sciences) have developed curricula in medical ethics that extend throughout the program of study -- including the clinical years and postgraduate internship and residency as well as the basic sciences years.

It may be tempting, when this sort of opportunity is presented, to allocate ethical theory to the pre-clinical years and to consign attention to application of theory to concrete clinical decisions to the clinical years of training. However, I am convinced that this would also be a mistake. The points I made above about the importance of establishing clinical relevance of ethical theory from the start dictate against beginning with a heavy dose of theory. Further, it has been my experience that a much greater appreciation of the thorniness and complexity of the dilemmas which arise in clinical practice comes about during the years of clinical training (when students face some of these dilemmas head-on for the first time) -- and, indeed, this appreciation increases still further during internship and residency when practitioners are first given full decision-making responsibility for cases. Thus practitioners at these points in their training may be ripe for further exploration of resources in ethical theory which could be brought to bear on the normative elements in these clinical decisions.

In view of these considerations, I propose the following structure for medical ethics teaching in connection with health professions training programs. This structure incorporates many elements of the curriculum we have developed in The University of Tennessee Inter-Campus Graduate Program in Medical Ethics; but it also includes some ideal elements (the value of which are seen on the basis of our ten years experience teaching medical ethics in this program) which have not yet been incorporated into the UT program.

Stage One -- Pre-Professional Years. At least one course in biomedical ethics should be required of every student (or, at the very least, strongly recommended) to provide a background upon which to build in teaching within the professional training program itself. This corresponds to the sort of background work in chemistry and biology that is currently required in the pre-professional years.

The ideal course at this level would begin with concrete examples of clinical cases (to establish relevance to clinical decision-making from the start, as well as to whet the students' appetite for ethical theory by demonstrating its usefulness as a tool for coming to grips with normative elements of clinical decisions). These early exercises would also serve to begin to make students aware of the ethical and value dimensions of clinical decisions [Objective 1] and would prompt an awareness of personal values and principles [Objective 2a]. The course should include a sound introduction to and exploration of a variety of ethical theories. However, these should not be studied in isolation. Rather, they should be regularly brought to bear on concrete clinical cases in order to probe their implications for clinical decisions [Objective 2c]. Thus the central teaching strategy employed in this course should be a "case method," although the discussion of cases should be pushed to the depth of considerable exploration of underlying conceptual issues [Objective 2e], points of ethical theory [Objective 2c], and elements of normative reasoning [Objective 2d]. General class discussion of cases will encourage students, not only to form reasoned conclusions about concrete cases [Objective 2f], but also to articulate both their conclusions and the reasoning behind them and to communicate these to fellow classmembers [Objective 3]. Written work in the course should also aim at communication of the process of reasoning out a conclusion in concrete cases. Ethical theory and the growing body of middle level literature in what we have come to call "medical ethics theory" can and should be referred to in defending one's conclusions, but essays and examinations should not become exercises in novice technical scholarship. Given the moral pluralism that characterizes our society, it is quite

11

likely that different students will reach diverse conclusions and/or support them by diverse patterns of reasoning. To further increase the variety of viewpoints represented, we have structured our preprofessional (undergraduate) medical ethics course (which is taught at UT-Knoxville) so that its enrollment includes (1) pre-health professions students in a wide variety of fields, (2) nursing students who have just begun clinical training, and (3) a general population of undergraduate students who bring the perspective of health care "consumer" to the issues. The contrasts between these viewpoints can further advance Objective 2c, as well as helping students become aware of their personal values and principles [Objective 2a] and prompting them to examine these critically [Objective 2b].

If no course dealing specifically with issues in biomedical ethics is available, a well-constructed course in ethical theory can advance many of these objectives (especially components of Objectives 2c, 2d, and 2e), though probably not as effectively as a course in some other area of applied ethics (e.g., business ethics, ethics in engineering) which makes use of a case method.

It is often suggested that pretty much any course in any humanities discipline will impart the same skills as a course in medical ethics, but I think our detailed list of objectives in section A can serve as a reference point to refute the claim. It may be true that many of the humanities disciplines can direct the student's attention to certain of the normative dimensions of clinical decisions and can guide him/her to grapple with these in one way or another. (They might, in other words, promote awareness of alternative points of view regarding values and ethical principles [one component of Objective 2c].) However, the skills of conceptual analysis [Objective 2e], probing patterns of reasoning [Objective 2d], critical analysis of alternative normative systems of thought [Objective 2b], and probing the implications of normative systems for concrete cases [Objectives 2c and 2f] are all associated uniquely with the discipline of philosophy.

NOTE on Constructing Case Studies. Our experience with the case study method has made it clear that the way case descriptions are constructed can make a vast difference in their effectiveness in prompting and guiding thought and discussion in the desired ways. The following are some guidelines that I drew up for use by students in our graduate concentration in medical ethics and by my colleagues who draw up case studies for conferences and classroom use:

SOME GUIDELINES FOR PREPARING
CASE STUDIES IN MEDICAL ETHICS

Three Primary Goals

(A) **Clinical Realism** -- to provide enough clinical informa-
    tion so that health professionals can gain a vivid and
    accurate grasp of the situation;

(B) **Ethical Thoroughness** -- to provide all the information
    needed for a sound discussion of the moral aspects of the
    situation;

(C) **Provocativeness** -- to present the information in a way
    that will prompt thought and discussion about the issue and
    will guide it in a sound and constructive direction.

1. The format of the case presentation should follow roughly
    the structure for presenting a clinical case. However, an
    exhaustive cataloge of data should **not** be attempted.
    Instead, the case description should be abbreviated by being
    restricted to "pertinent findings" (as is generally done in
    clinical case presentations).

2. In order to permit use of the case study by a wide variety
    of groups, explanation should be provided for technical
    terms and groups of findings.

3. Simplify, but don't **over** simplify! If too much or
    extraneous detail is included, the case may lack **focus**.
    On the other hand, if the case description focuses too nar-
    rowly on one specific moral issue, both clinical realism and
    ethical thoroughness may be lost.

4. Bring the case to a clear **decision-point**, at which a
    choice must be made. This prompts the reader to grapple
    with the issues and decide what s/he would do in this
    situation.

5. It may help to prompt focused thought to specify a **point
    of view** from which the issue should be considered -- e.g.,
    "Assume you are the physician...."

    If you want the situation to be considered from one specific
    point of view, cast the whole case description from this
    perspective.

    If you want several points of view to be taken into account,
    either (a) write variants of the case description from the

several viewpoints, or (b) write the case description from a neutral perspective, and specify the various viewpoints from which it is to be considered in the discussion questions.

6. Do not describe the outcome of the case! This invites the ethical fallacy of "Well, it came out okay in the end." No ethical theory holds that the test of right choices is actual outcome (since, if they did, the theory would be useless as a guide to choice -- which must always take place before the fact).

7. Groups discussing the case invariably ask about the actual outcome -- so you might describe it on a separate page (or else in informal accompanying materials intended for the discussion leader).

8. Whenever possible, describe a range of options.

    Such a list can serve several purposes:

    (a) The description of options may bring into focus key ethical elements of the situation not explicitly identified as such in the case description.

    (b) If options are phrased in terms of different ethical principles and theories, they may prompt the reader to relate the situation at hand to theoretical issues.

    (c) The list of options may widen the reader's horizon on thinking beyond the two or three choices that naturally occur to him or her.

    (d) The list may even spark the reader's imagination to come up with creative additional alternatives. [To allow for this, always include an open category -- "other (specify)."]

    List a wide range of choices. Don't hesitate to include a few that are clearly morally unacceptable. It may be a useful exercise to articulate why they are to be rejected.

9. Discussion questions are useful to guide thinking and discussion. Do not write a private agenda into the list of questions, however. Instead, encourage the reader to explore various perspectives on the issue.

10. Consider a multiple part case study if:

    (a) You want to present more than one perspective on an issue.

(b) You want to prompt re-thinking of an issue after an initial decision has been reached.

(c) You want to explore whether systematic variations of one element of the situation makes a difference to the ethical conclusions reached.

(d) You want to reveal the actual outcome of the situation at the end of the discussion.

For (a) and (c), it works best to give different versions of the case to different small groups, let them discuss it, and then let them compare notes after they have reached and announced their conclusions.

I want to underline the importance of describing cases in a way that brings the reader to a clear decision-point (item #4 on the list of guidelines). Many case studies in the literature focus on actions, practices, or outcomes (cf. guideline #6) which raise ethical issues; but they do not bother to probe the elements of the clinical decisions which led to these problematic features. If, as I have contended in section A above, the overall goal of medical ethics teaching in the clinical setting is to influence the process of clinical decision-making, it is crucial to focus on this process from the start; and thus it is essential, first, to include all the elements required to make a clinical decision and, second, to construct the case description in a way that prompts a reasoned and considered decision for the situation at hand.

Stage Two – Basic Medical Sciences Years. The focus and structure of medical ethics teaching here should be similar to that in the pre-professional years. In particular, the introduction should again focus on concrete clinical cases; and cases should remain a dominant focus throughout. If students have had the recommended prior course in biomedical ethics which provided them with a grounding in ethical theory and ethical-theory-oriented discussions of issues in biomedical ethics, then the reading material at this level can be drawn from the growing body of discussions of medical ethics issues to be found in the medical literature. However, it would be advisable to spend some time probing the points of ethical theory and medical ethics theory which form the (often unstated) background presuppositions of these essays. Not only can this lead to greater clarity of understanding about the heart of the debate, but it can also serve as a useful review of these elements of theory and of their implications for concrete clinical decisions. (If students have not had a prior course dealing with ethical theory, then the use of this literature will have to be supplemented with -- and perhaps even replaced by -- some material in ethical theory and exercises designed to develop the initial skills of critical analysis, conceptual analysis, and ethical reasoning in applying theory to concrete cases). All the same objectives dealt with in the preprofessional years would be aims here, as well. The goal would be to further develop and refine all these skills.

As in the pre-professional years, writing assignments should stress articulation and defense of the reasoning process involved in applying theory to concrete cases. One way to reinforce the point that analysis of the normative dimensions is an integral part of clinical decision-making is to introduce a device for structuring the analysis that is clearly related to those which the students are learning to employ for the assessment and management of the technical elements of clinical cases. One such device is the "Ethical Work-up" proposed by David C. Thomasma.[17] Another idea, not yet worked out as far as I know, is the suggestion made by a physician on the faculty at UTCHS that a section on "Ethical and Values Problems" be added to the Problem Oriented Medical Record. However, any of these devices would have to be supplemented with an extended additional explanation and defense of the sketchy account likely to result. The objectives of critical analysis and examination of reasoning require more thorough discussion than one typically finds entered into the medical record.

Stage Three -- Clinical Training Years. As I argued above, and as Ackerman also points out in his essay elsewhere in this volume,[18] if the objective of medical ethics teaching is to influence clinical decision-making and practice then it is absolutely essential that it be continued in significant forms during the clinical training years. Only in this way can the skills taught earlier be refined, reinforced, and brought to bear on clinical practice in a way that is likely to continue in later professional life.

The primary thrust of medical ethics teaching at this level should be to guide the student in his/her efforts to draw upon the skills and theoretical understanding which were developed in the two previous stages and apply them to decisions that arise in his/her own clinical practice.

The most effective means of achieving this would be for the medical ethics teacher and the practitioner-in-training to engage, together, in an extended analysis of clinical cases which the student is currently managing.

One mechanism for doing this which is employed in many institutions is to have periodic "Ethics Grand Rounds" conferences at which cases that have arisen in the institution are analyzed in detail by both the practitioner-in-training and clinical and/or medical ethics professionals. The chief problem here is that only a small number of cases can be dealt with in this way. What is needed is a mechanism which will focus some of the same sort of attention on a much larger number of cases.

Brody's suggestion of the model of "the good clinical consultant" may be thought to fill this need. However, I would maintain that at least one central feature of this model makes it unsuitable as a pattern for this stage of medical ethics teaching. Brody describes the feature I have in mind in this way:

> The good clinical consultant . . . is again a recognized expert in his own particular subspecialty. But his utility as a consultant is not based directly on his sharing of that expertise. Rather it is based on his willingness to answer a very specific question which arises out of a complex practical problem in clinical medicine. . . .
>
> The good clinical consultant . . . will answer the question that was asked briefly and to the point, indicating in general the background information on which he relied to reach his decision and indicating where the attending physician can proceed to find further information on the subject if desired.[19]

I see two problems with application of this model to medical ethics teaching at the level we are discussing. First, we cannot assume that the students are able to formulate specific questions to ask. If the two earlier stages of training described above have been effective, students at this level should have considerable skills in isolating the normative dimensions of clinical decisions; but there still might be significant normative issues in the case which they do not bring out for the consultant's analysis.

Second, and even more important, the goal of medical ethics teaching at this level is **not** to have an expert analyze the normative issues and offer definitive answers to those that are problematic. Rather, the aim is to guide the practitioner-in-training in conducting his/her own analysis of these elements and reaching answers on his/her own.[20]

I think a more satisfactory model for medical ethics teaching at this level would be the clinical case report conference or the working rounds. Selected cases which they are currently managing could be presented in some detail by the students, and they and the medical ethics teacher could work together to ferret out and analyze the normative dimensions of these cases.

However, although the focus on cases (here, actual cases from the students' current experience) should be primary, it should not be the whole task of medical ethics teaching at this level. Consideration of cases will inevitably give rise to conceptual puzzles and normative dilemmas which can be adequately addressed only by extended excursions into theoretical issues far beyond the scope that can be handled during hurried working conferences. Haavi Morreim responds to this need through short written pieces[21] -- a technique I also have sometimes used. However, given the severe limitations of the amount of material clinical students are likely to read and digest on their own, as well as the greater pedagogical effectiveness of face-to-face give-and-take, I would recommend that these occasions for teaching be supplemented by a periodic, on-going seminar at which these issues could be discussed in some depth. A regularly scheduled luncheon gathering might be a good way to bring this about. My colleagues and I in the UT Inter-Campus Graduate Program in Medical Ethics are currently developing a series of multimedia programs to help meet this need. A brief videotape, which includes a re-enactment of a typical clinical case and comments about it by one or more clinical and/or medical ethics professionals, is accompanied by a study guide booklet, which contains (1) exercises to prompt individual thought and small-group discussion analyzing the normative dimensions of the situation, (2) selected brief readings dealing with central conceptual and normative issues raised by the case, and (3) a carefully annotated bibliography for further study of these issues. These programs could be made available in clinical training centers, where interns and residents could work through them at their convenience -- either individually or in small groups. They might also be used under the guidance of a medical ethics teacher.

But, whatever format is employed, it is clear that some forum or other is needed at which the necessarily sketchy discussions of key issues during working sessions can be expanded and deepened. As I indicated above, my experience has been that these more extended discussions are welcomed by practitioners-in-training at this level. Their frustration at grappling with normatively thorny cases for the first time on their own responsibility makes them eager to acquire the theoretical resources that will enable them to unravel the normative complexities and dilemmas which they are encountering.

If it is possible to stimulate writing on the part of students at this level, it might usefully take the form of case reports in which selected cases from the student's own clinical experience are described and analyzed. These can, in turn, form a useful source of case descriptions to employ with other students in the earlier stages of training.

This format of medical ethics teaching can be applied throughout the years of clinical training -- i.e., during internships, residencies, and fellowships, as well as during the clinical years of medical school.

Stage Four -- Continuing Education for Practicing Professionals. It is at this stage that Brody's model of "the good clinical consultant" has its most suitable application. By this stage -- especially if they have been through the earlier stages of medical ethics training -- practitioners should have considerable skills in isolating key normative issues in the clinical decisions they face; and thus it can be left to them to take initiative to seek consultation on those which are especially troublesome. And, with regard to these, they may primarily be seeking suggested answers drawn from the expertise of professionals trained in clinical medical ethics rather than a less structured exercise in analyzing the normative dimensions of the decisions.

I would especially endorse one element in Brody's description of "the good clinical consultant:"

> Over time, by observing when the consultation requests that he receives seem appropriate and when they do not, the consultant will devise ways to interact more actively with his primary care colleagues, perhaps by involving himself in continuing education conferences at the hospital.[22]

In this way, the theoretical background can continue to be brought to the attention of practicing professionals. In my own work at the UT Memorial Research Center and Hospital in Knoxville, I have attempted to structure the monthly Ethics Grand Rounds conferences to cover certain key issues at regular intervals and in a format that combines analysis of a specific clinical case with some discussion of theoretical background material.

I believe we are now in a position to address the objections which were described early in section A of this essay (see p. 2 above). The first of these -- that philosophy has nothing distinctive to contribute to the skills of clinical decision-making and practice -- is the one that has been answered most fully in the course of our discussion. My list of specific objectives and skills indicates abundantly, I think, that philosophy has distinctive contributions to make. In order to dispute this, one must either refute my claim that clinical decisions contain essential normative components or else demonstrate alternative ways of imparting the skills of conceptual and normative analysis which are required to deal with these dimensions.

The **second** objection was that to put philosophy to the service of such practical goals as we have described represents a prostitution and impoverishment of the discipline. Caplan makes this point indirectly when he cites the two situations in which he himself was most efficacious in his work in a teaching hospital and points out that neither of them involved use of philosophical skills.[23] It is certainly true that many situations arise when all the philosopher in the clinical setting is called on to do is to exercise common sense -- aided by his or her perspective as one who does not take standard clinical procedures for granted. However, in other situations, issues will arise in clinical practice which pose genuine philosophical puzzles -- e.g., the concepts of a person and/or of rights as they figure in dilemmas concerning abortion, issues in philosophy of mind which figure in puzzles about patient competence, issues in epistemology in connection with questions about the degree of assurance to be sought in diagnosis or treatment selection. The analysis of these issues requires new steps in philosophical analysis and construction which go far beyond common sense. In addition, consideration of these puzzles may lead us to reconsider received doctrines in ethical theory, philosophy of mind, epistemology, and other areas of philosophy. We may discover that areas of philosophical scholarship are inadequate and impoverished as they stand, as demonstrated by their inability to deal with the issues which arise in clinical decisions; and, in turn, consideration of these issues may suggest new directions for revision of these received philosophical doctrines.

These same points can serve to answer the **third** of the objections: that applied philosophy is liable to amount to nothing more than a series of "techniques," without adequate attention to the fundamental background ruminations which form the heart and soul of the philosophical enterprise. This objection assumes that the medical ethics teacher will function as an ethics "answer man" (or woman) who is presented with dilemmas and spouts a definitive prescription without any explanation. But, as Brody points out, this is an inadequate description even of the model of a clinical consultant. Although the consultant is expected to provide a definite answer to the question posed, s/he is also expected to back this up with indications of the background theory on which the recommendation is based. Further, I have argued that the medical ethics teacher ought not to function even this closely to the "answer man" model -- with the possible exception of the stage of professional continuing education. Another image suggested by this objection is that of an "ethics cook book," in which simple techniques would be presented for reaching a definitive conclusion to any normative puzzle. However, the extreme reluctance of any philosopher to attempt to construct such a guide will be matched, I suspect, by a rejection of the notion by practitioners. "Cook book" ethics is likely to be as thoroughly scorned as is "cook book" clinical practice. As I have pointed out in the preceding discussion, there is abundant reason to integrate a focus on cases with extensive discussion of theoretical background material at every stage of the enterprise of clinical medical ethics teaching.

C. QUALIFICATIONS FOR CLINICAL MEDICAL ETHICS TEACHING

The objectives discussed in section A and the teaching strategies discussed in section B, in turn, help define the qualifications necessary for teaching clinical medical ethics. The sketch of qualifications that follows incorporates many of the elements we have sought to include in the UT Program of Graduate Studies in Philosophy with Concentration in Medical Ethics. In addition, besides the many and lengthy discussions of this question among the diverse faculty who designed this program and the recommendations of a distinguished panel of evaluation consultants who have advised us throughout the period of program development, I will draw from the results of a conference we held in 1979 at which medical educators and medical ethics professionals spent two full days discussing precisely this issues.[24]

1. **Personality Characteristics.** In his essay in this section, Howard Brody states: "I am convinced that certain personality characteristics, and the willingness to engage in sorts of activities and try the sorts of approaches that are infrequently encountered in academic philosophy or theology training, determine the success or failure of clinical ethics teaching much more frequently than do academic qualifications."[25] I wholeheartedly agree, and the group of medical educators who discussed this topic did as well. They listed as the prime qualification for clinical medical ethics teaching that the person be "mature and responsible, with an understanding of his/her role." Specific items which were brought out under this heading included: "a posture open to learn as well as to teach," "interpersonal skills in dealing with personnel in the clinical setting," "sensitivity to professional health care roles and responsibilities in the clinical setting," "a sense of personal professional goals and how these mesh with the objectives of the institution."

These traits can perhaps be taught to some extent (primarily through the influence of role models), but we have found that the most effective way to ensure them is in the process of selection of students to enter the program of study, supplemented by screening of students throughout their enrollment. Academic promise is certainly a prerequisite to success in a program of study aimed at producing clinical medical ethics teachers (for reasons we shall explain in a moment), but this is only a beginning. The standard academic measures must be supplemented by a serious attempt to determine the presence of these other requisite personal qualities.

2. **Academic Philosophy.** As Brody points out in connection with both his model of "the good basic science teacher" and "the good clinical consultant," recognized expertise in one's home discipline is also a **sine qua non** of respect and acceptance in health professions education. Before one can hope to apply philosophy to issues in clinical practice, one must have a thorough comprehension of the areas of philosophy to be applied. And, as I have indicated above, this is not restricted to the areas of ethical theory and medical ethics theory. Issues in epistemology, philosophy of mind, metaphysics, and other areas of the discipline also surface when clinical decisions are probed with rigor.

For these reasons, we at UT have chosen to structure our graduate program in medical ethics in terms of a concentration within a general program of graduate study in philosophy, rather than as a more limited alternative degree program or sub-discipline. Students concentrating in medical ethics at UT must fulfill all the requirements for the Ph.D. degree in philosophy, including preliminary examinations in the history of philosophy (ancient, medieval, and modern), contemporary epistemology and metaphysics, and ethical theory, a course requirement in philosophy of science, and a proficiency requirement in symbolic logic, as well as a comprehensive examination in medical ethics.

3. **Medical Ethics Theory.** The 1979 faculty conference listed as another important and needed qualification for medical ethics teaching: "knowledge of the major medical-ethics and medico-legal issues." In the UT program, we convey this through a series of seminars -- beginning with an entry-level survey course which introduces the case study method at the same time students are guided through a review of major components of the literature in medical ethics. Additional seminars are offered on selected topics and figures in the field, throughout the student's program of study; and seminars discussing background issues are co-ordinated with each clinical observation component of the program.

4. **Other Academic Disciplines.** The statement from the 1979 faculty conference quoted above in item #3 also indicated the importance of familiarity with certain other disciplines -- notably law. In the UT program, arrangements have been made for students to take courses in a number of other academic fields, including law, sociology, public health, history, economics, biology, psychology, and social work. Two of these areas have been found to be especially useful: (a) courses on the legal ramifications of clinical decisions and the underlying ethical issues, and

22

(b) a pair of courses in medical sociology which are available at our institution offers, not only a valuable review of the classic literature in this field, but also skills in clinical observation and analysis (especially related to interpersonal communications) which have proved extremely valuable to students.

5. Rudiments of Health Sciences. Without some knowledge of the terminology in which clinical cases are discussed and of the clinical details about them, medical ethics teachers will be unable to ferret out the normative issues when clinical cases are presented. Reliance on the clinical practitioners to point out and explain the ethical dimensions leaves the medical ethics professional wholly dependent on the level of skill which clinical practitioners have already developed in isolating the normative dimensions of clinical decisions. At best, this would severely hamper any progress in further developing objective #1 of section A above.

It is clear, then, that some degree of understanding of the rudiments of health sciences is a requisite qualification for effective medical ethics teaching in the clinical setting. At the first two stages of teaching described in Section B above, this might be limited to the background material relating to the case studies one uses in teaching -- but, even here, there is always the possibility that a knowledgeable student will introduce issues that go beyond the teacher's grasp. And, in the third and fourth stages of teaching described in section B -- at which clinical cases from the practitioner's present experience is the focus of attention -- a much wider range of technical knowledge is required.

The Hastings Center study group on applied ethics made the general recommendation that the equivalent of one year's study in the professional field in which one is working is required for effective teaching.[26] However, this is a difficult standard to interpret in connection with biomedical ethics teaching. Would a year's worth of courses in basic health sciences such as physiology be sufficient, or should a year of clinical study be chosen? But how can the person without any background in the basic health sciences hope to profit from clinical training? These questions are thorny indeed.

In the UT program, we have attempted to introduce the students to some rudiments of health sciences in the course of their program of study through a series of presentations, assignments, and readings which are integrated into our "Clinical Medical Ethics" courses. Elements we attempt to cover include:

(a) medical terminology -- This is taught by means of a well-structured programmed text which was designed for medical transcriptionists and allied health professionals.[27] Further reinforcement is provided by means of a series of word puzzles involving medical terminology,[28] as well as through specific questions in connection with case descriptions and clinical observations.

(b) **organ systems** -- This is taught with the aid of The Anatomy Coloring Book[29] and reinforced through case discussions.

(c) **disease entities** -- These are assigned to individual students for them to research and prepare a brief presentation to the group. Additional research assignments are often made in connection with case descriptions and clinical observations.

(d) **treatment modalities** -- Student-researched presentations and assigned research in the medical library or the several medical textbooks which we keep on hand in the department library[30] are supplemented by presentations by health professionals who work with our program.

(e) **the structure of clinical decision-making** -- Students are guided through clinico-pathological exercises, articles from the medical literature, and case reports they have observed and prompted to analyze the processes of reasoning involved.

(f) **research design and statistics** -- Sample research protocols, as well as research reports coupled with critical analyses of them (e.g., in letters to the editor of medical journals) are studied at the same time as guidelines for regulation of clinical research.

(g) **the structure of health care institutions and the domain of responsibility of the variety of personnel who staff them** -- This is taught through descriptions in the literature,[31] as well as by means of presentations by health care personnel and guided reflection on the student's own clinical observations.

(h) the history of health professional educa-
     tion -- Classic documents such as the
     Flexner report and descriptions of the devel-
     opment of educational structures[32] are com-
     bined with recent discussions of key elements
     of health professions education from current
     literature.[33]

(i) rudiments of the sciences of human func-
     tioning -- This is taught through readings
     in psycho-social dimensions of illness and
     care.[34]

Obviously, only the barest fundamentals of these areas can
be conveyed in the course of a program of graduate study in philosophy. Attempts to understand this material in greater depth
must continue throughout the professional career of a medical
ethics teacher. Our colleagues at UTCHS have found that one can
be most effective in clinical teaching if, rather than taking the
whole of medical science as one's province, one concentrates in
one or two specialty areas and attempts to gain a significant
competence there.[35]

     6. Clinical Familiarity. Since a good deal of the
teaching we have described takes place in the clinical setting,
it is vital that medical ethics teachers be familiar with the
realities of clinical practice. Even in teaching at the first
two stages outlined in section B above, an understanding of
clinical realities and their impact on decision-making and practice is essential to effective teaching.

     To this end, the UT program of graduate study includes an
extensive structured series of clinical observations -- (a) beginning during the first two years of study with attendance at case
conferences and hospital rounds at the teaching hospital in
Knoxville, (b) continuing with a two-month clinical internship at
a state psychiatric hospital, (c) continuing further with the
intensive ten-week Clinical Practicum at UTCHS in Memphis, which
consists of extended observation of health care procedures in a
wide range of settings at more than a dozen clinical sites,
including surgery, psychiatry, cancer care (adult and pediatric),
intensive care (adult and perinatal), family medicine, internal
medicine, pediatrics, emergency room services, spinal cord injury
services, respiratory disease treatment, and community medicine,
and (d) with an intensive clinical observation in a specific area
of the student's choice.

     In all of these varied clinical experiences, observation is
combined with seminars, reading assignments and faculty supervision in an attempt to train the students to analyze clinical
decisions and then to employ philosophical skills and knowledge

25

to address these issues in a way that will be readily understand-able and helpful to both clinical health services professionals and academic philosophers alike.

7. **Training in Teaching.** One woeful gap in most post-graduate programs in philosophy is lack of attention to training in teaching. In the UT program, we attempt to provide this training in several ways: through instruction in the case study method and other aspects of teaching, through supervised employment of graduate students as assistants in our teaching efforts -- including both our undergraduate course and our clinical teaching activities, as well as in public service presentations of issues in medical ethics.

Prepared with these qualifications, graduates of the program are able to carry out the teaching strategies described in section B and, by means of them, achieve the objectives described in section A.

FOOTNOTES

[1]For a critical view of the role of the ethicist as consultant, see Arthur Caplan's essay, "Can Applied Ethics Be Effective in Health Care and Should It Strive to Be?", **ETHICS** 93 (January, 1983), pp. 111-121; this volume, pp. 129-141. By contrast, John Robertson argues that a moral duty exists and a legal duty may be emerging on the part of the physician to consult with medical ethics advisors on thorny cases. See his essay, "Clinical Medical Ethics: Rights and Duties in Ethics Consultations," this volume, pp. 67-79.

[2]Caplan views this as the arena in which medical ethics can make the most effective contribution. See Caplan, op. cit.

[3]Caplan raises such questions in several ways in his essay in this section. See Caplan, this volume, especially pp. 131-132.

[4]This is one component of what Caplan calls the "engineering model" of bioethics.

[5]See pp. 19-21 below for the summary replies to these objections.

[6]Ackerman, this volume, p. 144-145. See also, Terrence Ackerman, "What Bioethics Should Be," **THE JOURNAL OF MEDICINE AND PHILOSOPHY** 5 (September 1980), 261.

[7]Edmund D. Pellegrino and David C. Thomasma, **A PHILOSOPHICAL BASIS OF MEDICAL PRACTICE** (New York: Oxford University Press, 1981), pp. 224-225.

[8]Eric J. Cassell, **THE HEALER'S ART: A NEW APPROACH TO THE DOCTOR-PATIENT RELATIONSHIP** (Philadelphia: J.B. Lippincott Co., 1976), p. 87.

[9]Ibid., p. 109.

[10]Some medical ethics theorists may be lured into this same mistake. See, for example, the "medical indications policy" proposed by Paul Ramsey in his **ETHICS AT THE EDGES OF LIFE** (New Haven: Yale University Press, 1978).

[11]In formulating this and the other objectives which I list in this section, I am indebted to Howard Brody's fine textbook **ETHICAL DECISIONS IN MEDICINE**, 2nd edition (Boston: Little, Brown and Company, 1981), pp. xv-xvii. I would also agree wholeheartedly with Brody's list of "Not Objectives":

After completing this book, the student will **not** be able to:

1. Recite a set of rules of proper medical conduct, the application of which will assure that one does the ethical thing in any instance.

2. State an ethical decision-making method that, for any specific case, will yield one and only one "right" answer as to the ethical thing to do.

3. Cite a code of ethics that will guide one's behavior in all problematic cases.

4. Discuss some aspect of medical law, and state how the law would view any action taken in a specific case. (p. xvii)

[12]On this notion, see R. M. Hare, **THE LANGUAGE OF MORALS** (London: Oxford University Press, 1952), pp. 68-69. By using this notion, I do not mean to endorse all aspects of Hare's interpretation of it, nor his analysis of the nature of moral judgments or the logic of moral reasoning.

[13]See John Rawls, **A THEORY OF JUSTICE** (Cambridge: Harvard University Press, 1971), pp. 20ff., 48-51.

[14]Pellegrino and Thomasma, op. cit., p. 135.

[15]For a similar statement on this point, see Howard Brody, "Teaching Clinical Ethics: Models for Consideration," this volume, p. 35.

[16]Ibid., pp. 32-35.

[17]David C. Thomasma, "Training in Medical Ethics: An Ethical Work-Up," **FORUM ON MEDICINE** 1 (December 1978), pp. 33-36.

[18]Ackerman, this volume, pp. 160-162.

[19]Brody, this volume, pp. 38-39.

[20]On this point, see the discussion by E. Haavi Morreim, "The Philosopher in the Clinical Setting," **THE PHAROS** (Winter 1983), especially pp. 4-5.

[21]Ibid., p. 3.

[22]Brody, this volume, p. 39.

[23]Caplan, this volume, pp. 129-131.

[24]See also, L.B. Cebik, "The Professional Role and Clinical Education of the Medical Ethicist," ETHICS IN SCIENCE AND MEDICINE 6 (1979), pp. 115-121.

[25]Brody, this volume, p. 32.

[26]THE TEACHING OF ETHICS IN HIGHER EDUCATION: A REPORT BY THE HASTINGS CENTER (Hastings-on-Hudson, NY: Institute of Society, Ethics, and the Life Sciences, 1980), pp. 63-65.

[27]Genevieve Love Smith and Phyllis E. Davis, MEDICAL TERMINOLOGY: A PROGRAMMED TEXT, 4th ed. (New York: John Wiley & Sons, 1981).

[28]Susan M. Sparks and Joyce L. Hayman, WORD GAMES FOR HEALTH PROFESSIONALS (New York: American Journal of Nursing Company, Volume I - 1978, Volume II - 1979).

[29]Wynn Kapit and Lawrence M. Elson, THE ANATOMY COLORING BOOK (New York: Canfield Press/Barnes & Noble, 1977).

[30]Some books we have found especially useful for this purpose include: Robert Berkow, (Editor-in-Chief), THE MERCK MANUAL OF DIAGNOSIS AND THERAPY, 14th edition (Rahway, N.J.: Merck & Co., 1982); Frances K. Widman, PATHOLOGY: HOW DISEASE HAPPENS (Boston: Little, Brown, 1978); William Boyd & Huntington Sheldon, AN INTRODUCTION TO THE STUDY OF DISEASE 7th edition (New York: Lea & Febiger, 1977); Elmer L. DeGowin and Richard L. DeGowin, BEDSIDE DIAGNOSTIC EXAMINATION, 3rd edition (New York: Macmillan, 1976); PATIENT CARE FLOW CHART MANUAL, 1980 edition (Darien, CT: Patient Care Publications, 1980); Donald M. Vickery and James F. Fries, TAKE CARE OF YOURSELF: A CONSUMER'S GUIDE TO MEDICAL CARE (Reading, MA: Addison-Wesley, 1976); PHYSICIANS' DESK REFERENCE (Oradell, NJ: Medical Economics Company); AMA DRUG EVALUATIONS, 4th edition (New York: John Wiley & Sons, 1980); and Harold M. Silverman and Gilbert I. Simon, THE PILL BOOK: THE ILLUSTRATED GUIDE TO THE MOST PRESCRIBED DRUGS IN THE UNITED STATES (New York: Bantam Book, 1979).

[31]For example, Judith Nierenberg and Florence Janovic, THE HOSPITAL EXPERIENCE: A COMPLETE GUIDE TO UNDERSTANDING AND PARTICIPATING IN YOUR OWN CARE (Indianapolis: Bobbs-Merrill, 1978); I. Donald Snook, Jr., HOSPITALS: WHAT THEY ARE AND HOW THEY WORK (Rockville, MD: Aspen Systems Corporation, 1981); Michael Crichton, FIVE PATIENTS (New York: Bantam Books, 1971); Philip R. Lee and Carol Emmott, "Health Care: Health Care System," THE ENCYCLOPEDIA OF BIOETHICS (Warren T. Reich, Editor-in-Chief) (New York: Macmillan/Free Press, 1978), pp. 610-619; Alain C. Enthoven, "What Medical Care Is and Isn't," in HEALTH PLAN: THE ONLY PRACTICAL SOLUTION TO THE SOARING COST

OF MEDICAL CARE (Reading, MA: Addison-Wesley, 1980); Eliot Freidson, PROFESSIONAL DOMINANCE: THE SOCIAL STRUCTURE OF MEDICAL CARE (New York: Atherton Press, 1970); Paul Starr, THE SOCIAL TRANSFORMATION OF AMERICAN MEDICINE (New York: Basic Books, 1982).

[32]Carnegie Commission on Higher Education, HIGHER EDUCATION AND THE NATION'S HEALTH: POLICIES FOR MEDICAL AND DENTAL EDUCATION (New York: McGraw-Hill, 1970); Abraham Flexner, MEDICAL EDUCATION IN THE UNITED STATES AND CANADA: A REPORT TO THE CARNEGIE FOUNDATION FOR THE ADVANCEMENT OF TEACHING (New York: The Carnegie Foundation for the Advancement of Teaching, 1910).

[33]Edmund D. Pellegrino, "Medical Education," ENCYCLOPEDIA OF BIOETHICS, op. cit., pp. 863-870; Charles L. Bosk, FORGIVE AND REMEMBER: MANAGING MEDICAL FAILURE (Chicago: The University of Chicago Press, 1979); Wendy Carlton, "IN OUR PROFESSIONAL OPINION . . .": THE PRIMACY OF CLINICAL JUDGMENT OVER MORAL CHOICE (Notre Dame, IN: University of Notre Dame Press, 1978); Ludwig W. Eichna, "Medical School Education, 1975-1979: A Student's Perspective," THE NEW ENGLAND JOURNAL OF MEDICINE 303 (September 25, 1980), pp. 727-734; Emily Mumford, INTERNS: FROM STUDENTS TO PHYSICIANS (Cambridge: Harvard University Press, 1970); Samuel Shem, THE HOUSE OF GOD (New York: Dell, 1980).

[34]See especially, Jurrit Bergsma and David C. Thomasma, HEALTH CARE: ITS PSYCHOSOCIAL DIMENSIONS (Pittsburgh: Duquesne University Press, 1982); Miriam Siegler and Humphrey Osmond, PATIENTHOOD: THE ART OF BEING A RESPONSIBLE PATIENT (New York: Macmillan, 1979); Martin R. Lipp, RESPECTFUL TREATMENT: THE HUMAN SIDE OF MEDICAL CARE (New York: Harper and Row, 1977). Among the most effective devices to convey this dimension of illness are first-person accounts of illness, especially including: Norman Cousins, ANATOMY OF AN ILLNESS AS PERCEIVED BY THE PATIENT (New York: W.W. Norton, 1979); Michael Halberstram and Stephen Lesher, A CORONARY EVENT (New York: Popular Library, 1976); Martha Weinman Lear, HEARTSOUNDS (New York: Simon and Schuster, 1980); Robert and Suzanne Massie, JOURNEY (New York: Warner Books, 1973); Susan Sontag, ILLNESS AS METAPHOR (New York: Farrar, Strauss, and Girou, 1977).

[35]Ackerman, this volume, pp. 161-162.

TEACHING CLINICAL ETHICS: MODELS FOR CONSIDERATION

Howard Brody

Over the past 10 years a number of articles and several books have been devoted to the teaching of medical ethics in the clinical setting. Although some of these works make claims to comprehensiveness, the majority of these papers do not even attempt to give a complete overview of the subject and merely call attention to one or more particular features of clinical ethics teaching which may be useful for those designing teaching programs to attend to more closely. When, in the literature to date, a comprehensive overview has been promised, the promise has seldom been fulfilled.

The paper I will present will follow in the more modest tradition and make no claims to completeness. There are a number of reasons for this. First, I do not believe that we have been engaged in this activity long enough to claim to have a thorough knowledge of the possible range of approaches to teaching strategies. This is true especially because we have been relatively neglectful of the techniques of evaluation and have seldom measured the effectiveness of the teaching we have done or the actual impact or the lack of impact it has had on the clinical setting where it has been carried out. Second, my comments will necessarily be based in large part upon the nine years experience we have had in clinical ethics teaching at Michigan State University; and most people involved in such programs will readily acknowledge that which strategies are most successful and which objectives are most attainable depends heavily upon the peculiarities of the institutional setting and the past history of the program itself. For example, within the last two to three years we have been rethinking many of our approaches to teaching ethics, not because the earlier approaches were necessarily wrong, but in fact because their existence changed the institution in ways that allow us now to aim at different goals. Any advice from us would be of very limited use to an ethics teaching program in a different institution which did not share a similar history. Third, largely because of time constraints I will restrict my comments to the teaching of medical ethics to medical students and medical house officers. Some of what I say will have relevance for the continuing medical education for practicing physicians in medical ethics. However I will leave undiscussed the very interesting and challenging concerns involved in teaching nursing ethics and clinical ethics teaching for other health professionals besides physicians.

It is customary to begin the discussion of clinical ethics teaching by noting the qualifications that are to be required of those who would engage in the practice. I wish to avoid this subject almost entirely, largely because I am convinced that certain personality characteristics, and the willingness to engage in these sorts of activities and try the sorts of approaches that are infrequently encountered in academic philosophy or theology training, determine the success or failure of clinical ethics teaching much more frequently than do academic qualifications. The concern that we will degrade the quality of our enterprise if we pay insufficient attention to academic credentials is not totally misplaced; but on the other hand I believe the much more likely danger is that we will render ourselves totally irrelevant to the clinical setting in which we ought to be working if we engage in too much nit-picking over credentials. At this point I will simply state that I believe it necessary (but not sufficient) that anyone teaching clinical medical ethics have a thorough grounding in general ethical theory based on either a philosophical or a theological approach to ethics. I freely acknowledge that we could easily spend the rest of this conference arguing about what exactly that means; so I will now proceed instead to suggesting what personal characteristics and practical strategies ought to accompany that background expertise.

I would like to approach the body of my talk by describing three models, the consideration of which may prove useful for improving the quality of clinical ethics teaching. The first model is aimed at depicting certain important characteristics of the medical student or house officer who is supposed to be the recipient of our teaching - characteristics which, I am afraid, have often been neglected in the literature on the subject. The second two models are intended to highlight ways in which medical ethics can learn from successful clinical teaching in other aspects of medicine. These models have been selected specifically to suggest teaching strategies and teaching objectives. I hope that I need not remind a philosophically sophisticated audience that when one compares a model to the original object, the disanalogies are as important as the analogies. I will take it for granted, for example, that when I use the model of a skilled cardiology consultant in order to highlight some possible teaching modes, no one will make the mistake of thinking that I am arguing that the field of medical ethics is a subspecialty of clinical medicine analogous to cardiology as a subspecialty of internal medicine.

The first model I wish to describe is a somewhat overdrawn sketch of the emotional reactions of the typical medical student to the medical education process. I will follow the suggestion of the popular novel, **THE HOUSE OF GOD** - why this book comes to mind may be more obvious later - and call our typical medical student BMS (the universal designation for all medical students currently enrolled in the "Best Medical School," of which, by common consent of students and faculty, there are some 40 or 50 existing in this country). BMS has been carefully selected for medical school enrollment as a result of a cutthroat competition process and as a result of having achieved phenomenal success in almost every enterprise which he has attempted in the course of his 22 years. That is, BMS has been carefully selected to have had the least possible experience in dealing with failure, his own inherent limitations, his incompetence in any field of knowledge or skill, and the natural emotional reactions which follow from the recognition of these. With this gross deficiency of potential coping skills, and almost no emotional support structure to assist him in responding to this deficiency, BMS is now embarked on a life experience which without too much exaggeration can be characterized as progressive incompetence. BMS begins this experience with the first of his basic science courses, perhaps anatomy. He is told at the very beginning of this course by his instructors that he knows almost no anatomy; and that in fact even if he successfully completes the course with honors he will still know almost no anatomy, since the fund of knowledge of this basic science is so vast that there is no conceivable way that more than a small fraction of it could be included in the already crowded medical curriculum. But BMS perseveres and by applying himself studiously gradually begins to feel that he knows something of this particular subject. As soon as this emotionally gratifying point is reached he is rudely kicked out of the anatomy nest and assigned to begin his next course, perhaps in physiology. Again he is told how woefully ignorant he is in physiology; how vast the field of physiology is; and how it is impossible to teach him more than a few scattered remnants of this knowledge in the short time available in the medical course. In this way BMS progresses from one to another of his basic science courses during the first two years of medical school. He begins each course, as it were, lashed to a stake set out in a desert with the hot sun of his incompetence beating down upon him and the thirst-quenching waters of competence lying far below at his feet. Slowly the waters begin to rise and he begins to have hope that eventually they will reach his parched lips. Then, as soon as the waters reach that level, someone abruptly pulls the plug, the waters are drained away and the stake is moved on to the next desert so that he can begin the process all over again.

Finally BMS has completed his first two years of medical training and has signaled this accomplishment by passing Part One of the National Boards - which "passing" means incidentally that he has failed to answer correctly somewhere between one-third and two-thirds of the questions asked in the entire exam. He is now ready to begin demonstrating a more sophisticated level of incompetence as he begins his clinical rotations. He shows up for the first day of his clinical clerkship, perhaps in internal medicine, feeling that he cannot possibly remember all that he has learned about the basic history and physical exam, let alone make any sense of the patient's symptoms and determine how to diagnose and treat the illness. It is not unlikely that the house staff and the nurses with whom he has to interact will find a variety of ways to remind him continually of the vast gaps in his knowledge. But again BMS perseveres and again after ten or twelve weeks he is finally starting to sense a few gratifying glimmers of competence shining through on the horizon. Now, of course, he is forced to leave internal medicine and go on to pediatrics, where BMS has to ask a whole different set of questions in taking the history, he has to consider a different set of illnesses in a differential diagnosis, he has to consider a whole different scale of dosages in prescribing medications, and he has to go off to a different part of the hospital where he does not even know where the bathroom or the coffee pot is located. And again the process is repeated as BMS goes from one to another of his required clerkships completing his last two years of medical school.

If BMS elects to go into a primary specialty or to take a rotating internship upon graduation he can look forward to one more year of this progressive incompetence cycle to continue, for a total of five years of his adult life having been spent in this sort of activity. He may then look forward to gradual acquisition of some real and justified sense of basic competence in his chosen area as he moves on into the second and third years of his residency training. On the other hand, if he goes into one of the surgical specialties or some training requiring a more extended period of residency, it may well be a total of seven or eight years before BMS finally begins to have good grounds for feeling that he is becoming somewhat competent. As BMS finally moves on into clinical practice he need no longer face the day to day, constant and glaring awareness of incompetence that was his experience as a medical student and intern. However this does not mean that the specter of incompetence and failure has been banished from his psyche. For most physicians it lurks somewhere in the background, as BMS recalls that only one momentary failure of attention or one isolated deficiency in his medical knowledge could spell disaster for a patient and the irreparable loss of his reputation among his peers.

The saga of BMS may appear to be somewhat at odds with the picture of medical education that has been presented in the literature on clinical ethics teaching. In much of this literature, pomposity, arrogance and inappropriate generalization of expertise, rather than the incompetence, fear of failure, and emotional vulnerability are taken to be characteristic of the affective landscape of clinical medicine. But that the model does in fact have some applicability is suggested, among other things, by the success and attention given to the novel, **THE HOUSE OF GOD**, and the surrealistic picture that it presents of a respected teaching hospital. (For purposes of education in the medical humanities, it is useful to discuss this novel with senior medical students and house officers as a representative work of satire and parody as applied to medicine. But one encounters a great deal of difficulty in doing this, because many medical students and house officers insist that the world depicted in the novel is not recognizable at all as satire, but in fact appears to them to be starkly realistic.) The medical house officers who populate the House of God have evolved a set of bizarre defense mechanisms to survive in that world, despite the cost that they pay in terms of their inhumanity both to themselves and to their patients. One must then ask what exactly is the emotional threat that prompted the formation of such desperate and primitive defense mechanisms in the first place. And when one asks that question, the saga of BMS does not seem too far off the mark as a portrayal of the emotional atmosphere that accompanies the medical education process.

The model of the emotional state of the average medical student just presented naturally has important implications for clinical ethics teaching. It suggests a series of questions that could be asked about a typical medical ethics teaching program. Is the ethics teaching program, for example, dealing with the ethical issues that arise for the students in their daily lives as a result of their vulnerable and incompetent status, as well as the more standard ethical issues that appear in the usual anthologies? (Whether the medical student should introduce himself to the patient as "Doctor" is only one obvious example.) Is the ethics teaching program helping the students to become consciously aware of their emotional reactions to their surroundings and the positive as well as the negative defense mechanisms they might evolve to deal with these? Or is the medical ethics teaching program reinforcing the dominant mood of clinical institutions, where denial of one's emotional vulnerability is frequently seen as the hallmark of "professionalism"? Is the ethics teaching program searching for ways to change the emotional atmosphere and the real pressures of the medical education system, wherever this may be practical? Or is the medical ethics course presented as simply one more arena in which the students' incompetence can be demonstrated before themselves, their fellow students and the faculty?

The teacher of clinical ethics about to begin a teaching program may try to ask questions such as these and to be guided in his efforts by the answers. He may naturally ask how he can make sure that the ethics program will be a positive rather than a negative experience for the medical students and house staff. He naturally might then be asked where in the existing world of clinical education he can find some examples of positive teaching experiences and strategies, which diminish the students' emotional concern over their incompetence by giving them, in a way that contributes to their self-esteem, some positive knowledge and skills which will be of real use to them as medical professionals. I will suggest that two models may serve our developing ethics instructor very well here; the model of the good basic science teacher and the model of the good clinical consultant. The ethics instructor who can guide his behavior by the first of these models will find that he will be especially effective in the first two years of medical school; the instructor who can best adapt to the second model will find that he will be welcomed especially by third and fourth year medical students and house officers.

The two clinical teaching models balance the first model, that of the "progressive incompetence" view of medical education, in an important way. Taken alone, the first model seems to place clinical ethics teaching in a bind. Either ethics instruction can be fully integrated into the body of medical education, and so become one more hurdle in BMS's obstacle course; or it can be kept carefully distinct from that process, and so be perceived by the students and house staff as forming no part of their professional development. If BMS's pilgrim's progress were in fact one uninterrupted vale of tears, this depressing dilemma would be an accurate overview. But the chances are very good that BMS did occasionally find solace in some positive learning experiences, which imparted really practical knowledge and skills in a way that served to enhance BMS's self-esteem as a developing professional. The two models I will present are intended to help the ethics instructor selectively identify the most positive elements in medical teaching and hence to avoid the all-or-none dilemma.

Let us consider first the model of the good basic science teacher. (It is important to emphasize here that I do not mean the model of the average or typical basic science teacher; unfortunately my nonquantifiable impression is that "good" individuals are quite rare among medical school faculties.) This teacher (let us say, for example, a physiologist) is a skilled investigator in his own parent discipline and is fully competent to replicate himself as a physiologist by the training of graduate students who will eventually become skilled investigators in physiology. This physiologist, however, has chosen willingly and we hope enthusiastically not to devote all his time to research and teaching of graduate students but instead to spend some of his time teaching students in a different profession who will never be his colleagues. He does this (we hypothesize optimistically) out of genuine respect for the practitioners of this other profession, medicine, equal to the respect that he holds for his fellow physiologists. Our physiologist is fully aware that a physician who does not know any physiology will be a poor physician, but he is equally aware of the many other objects that a physician must master and the limited time in the medical curriculum that he has to learn them. Our physiologist therefore has thoughtfully identified the minimal content from his own discipline that one needs to know in order to practice medicine effectively. His ability to do this implies that he has somehow achieved a knowledge of

36

medical practice which is extremely rare among those who now teach basic science in medical schools. Our physiologist then seeks to organize this material and present it in an interesting and compelling fashion to his medical students. He is willing, in planning his lectures, to be guided by their needs as future practitioners of a profession different from his own. He specifically avoids the temptation, all too common among professors in universities generally, to design his lectures as if he expected one of his colleagues to drop in at the back of the room and eavesdrop at any time, and was fearful that his professional colleague might be insufficiently impressed with the quality and erudition of his lecture. Our ideal physiologist has sufficient self-confidence not to care what his lecture will sound like to his department chairman, so long as it gets the essential points across to the medical students who are depending on him for their education.

When we dig deeper and ask just how this physiologist decided what, out of the entire field of physiology, he ought to include in his medical school course, we approach the limits of the analogy between basic science teaching and ethics teaching, and hence come to the point where the most challenging questions can be asked. The average basic science teacher (not the good one) makes this decision by noting that medical students will never become research physiologists and thus, supposedly, have no need for any understanding of scientific methodology or theory; so the lectures should be instead crammed as full as possible with factual knowledge. These "rat facts," which fit so nicely into the multiple-choice test format, do not in the end appear to be all that terrible; practicing physicians remember hardly any of what they were taught in physiology and yet still seem to know enough practical physiology to take reasonable care of their patients. But the emphasis on "rat facts" to the exclusion of other modes of instruction is largely responsible for the well-deserved label of anti-intellectualism with which physicians as a group are often branded; it helps to explain why so few physicians can read a journal article in a critical and thoughtful manner; and it accounts for why physiology class is not any fun. Now this is not the sort of mistake that the ethics instructor is likely to make; even if he knows the years in which Kant was born and died, he is not going to be tempted to make the students memorize them. But how much theoretical language is necessary as background knowledge; and how much of medical ethics can be presented in the form of packaged conclusions, how much as opposing arguments, and how much as a process of inquiry, poses the most vexing questions. The good basic science teacher has spent a good deal of time deciding how much of his course is teaching physiology and how much is about teaching to think physiologically; but the extent to which his answers will be helpful to the clinical ethics instructor is not immediately obvious. It seems to me that the question is at least worth posing in this fashion; I see no value in assuming at the start that the ethics instructor has nothing to learn from the basic science teacher and thereby cutting off further inquiry.

The other model our ethics instructor may wish to emulate is the model of the good clinical consultant. My judgment (again based on very limited data) is that this individual fortunately is more commonly encountered than our ideal basic science teacher. The good clinical consultant, whose arrival is greeted with enthusiasm by senior medical students, house officers and attending faculty, is again a recognized expert in his own particular subspecialty. But his utility as a consultant is not based directly on his sharing of that expertise. Rather it is based on his willingness to answer a very specific question which arises out of a complex practical problem in clinical medicine. (This has important implications for the statement sometimes heard from philosophers who teach ethics in clinical settings that they are very careful to discuss and analyze the issues in detail, but also to warn people in advance that they are not to be expected to give final answers. The clinical consultant who advertises in advance that he will not give answers can be guaranteed a great deal of leisure and relatively few consultations.)

When the clinical consultant gives an answer to the question that was posed, the physicians primarily responsible for that patient's care assume that the answer given has been informed by the vast expertise of that consultant in his subspecialty field. But what they are seeking from that consultant is not that expertise per se but rather the ability to focus that expertise on the particular problem at hand. Let us suppose for example that a patient who is otherwise a poor surgical candidate has suffered several attacks over a few months which have been diagnosed as the consequences of gallstones plugging the common bile duct. The attending physician is struggling with the issue of how likely these attacks are to recur frequently in the future so that the risks of surgery for this patient can be weighed against the risks of recurrent episodes of gallstone disease. To assist in answering this question, a gastroenterologist is consulted. If this gastroenterologist then proceeds to adorn the patient's chart with a four-page treatise on the physiology of gallbladder contractility, his efforts will not be at all appreciated by the primary physician, regardless of the fact that everything stated in the consultation note is absolutely true and that the organization of the material may in fact be nothing short of brilliant. This consultant has answered at great length a question which was not asked and hence has proved useless in the clinical setting.

The good clinical consultant, by contrast, will answer the question that was asked briefly and to the point, indicating in general the background information on which he relied to reach his decision and indicating where the attending physician can proceed to find further information on the subject if desired. The good clinical consultant furthermore has helped to reassure the attending physician that his advice really is pertinent to this particular patient's problem by the fact that he has been willing to see, talk to and examine this patient and has also indicated his willingness to follow the patient throughout the remainder of the hospital course if that should be desirable. In some cases this means that the consultant has gained crucial information directly from the patient which he could not otherwise have obtained. However, in many cases, what this probably signifies is merely that the presence of the consultant has been emotionally reassuring to the primary physician, who can now go ahead and do what he has to do with the comforting knowledge that someone else of equal or greater authority is behind him.

Of course the notion that the consultant will meekly answer whatever question is posed to him by the primary physician cannot be accepted without qualification. It is the willingness to answer a practical question posed within the context of direct patient care that gives the consultant his first entry into this particular clinical setting. But naturally after being consulted dozens of times for cases of earwax, the otolaryngologist may feel that he is not well serving the general educational function that he owes to the community of primary care physicians. Over time, by observing when the consultation requests that he receives seem appropriate and when they do not, the consultant will devise ways to interact more actively with his primary care colleagues, perhaps by involving himself in continuing education conferences at the hospital. He will use these opportunities to educate the attending physicians further on what questions his expertise allows him to answer and what questions are really outside his realm and should best be referred to other authorities. In the process, of course, the consultant may well have been educated by the attending physicians on how he himself ought to define his special area of expertise. The very frequency of certain problems for which he originally showed little enthusiasm, or the very perplexing nature of those problems for the attending physicians, may have forced him to define more broadly his area of concern and to seek to expand his knowledge into those problem areas.

These models are worthy of consideration by the ethics instructor because they demonstrate how despite the staggering amount of information that must be assimilated by physicians in training, and the often ego-shattering emotional climate in which this information is accumulated and imparted, mechanisms have evolved for transmitting this information in an educationally helpful and practically useful manner. The value of these teaching models is unfortunately often driven home by comparing them with the more negative models that medical students and house officers encounter all too frequently. In a stereotypical university teaching center, for every one of the ideal basic professors we have depicted, there are several who are only too ready to ridicule the medical students by reminding them that the very brightest in their class does not even approach that professor's dumbest graduate student in their grasp of the basic science material. For every one of the good clinical consultants we have described, the student and house officer is likely to encounter several attending physicians who are only too happy to deride them during morning rounds for not remembering what the patient's chloride level was three days ago or for not having read the research report on the patient's disease which will appear in next week's issue of the NEW ENGLAND JOURNAL OF MEDICINE.

The ethics instructor, having reviewed these models, may acknowledge that he can perceive many useful analogies between good ethics teaching and good teaching of other clinical subjects. However he might reasonably object that I have given him no guidance in the equally important problem of identifying the disanalogies between the content and skills that should be taught as part of medical ethics and the content and skills of other aspects of clinical medicine. It is crucial that this instructor understand where the models break down and where he must look to the intellectual integrity of the discipline of ethics itself, rather than other examples of clinical teaching, to know how to proceed. In this regard the comments of Arthur Caplan and others on the appropriate ways of conceptualizing applied ethics in medicine are certainly indispensible tools for the ethics instructor. As might be inferred by some of Caplan's work, the analysis of what it means to do applied ethics in medicine is most useful when it is aimed at determining why clinical ethicists succeed in some activities that they attempt and fail in others, and in what sorts of practical day-to-day activities the medical ethicists ought to engage. Beyond this I am not sure how far this debate can be successfully carried without turning into a fruitless nondebate. It often seems that the arguments over applied ethics are disagreements more over practical emphasis than over the nature of medical ethics itself, since it often turns out that the supposed positions argued for by the supposed disputants in the supposed debate are in no way logically incompatible. (Where they are logically incompatible, the problem seems to arise from disagreements over general ethical theory which cannot and ought not to be resolved with reference to medical ethics only.) Regarding one target of the argument on applied medical ethics -- the inflexible philosopher who stubbornly tries to fit every complex medical issue into his own pet metaethical theory -- I am not sure where such individuals are to be found; perhaps our ethics program has been singularly blessed with the absence of anyone answering this description. Furthermore there seems to be some danger that the champions of applied ethics will repeat the mistake that their immediate predecessors (now derided as the "armchair ethics crowd") attributed to the physicians -- thinking that immersion in medical dilemmas on a day-to-day basis gives them sort of privileged access to important facts which are unique to the sphere of medical care.

There is good reason to believe on the contrary that the problems of doing medical ethics in a meaningful way are in many cases simply the problems generally of doing ethics in the real world when one is dealing with complex social issues. And the problems of teaching ethics are in many ways simply the problems of how to achieve good teaching, especially in the clinical setting, but elsewhere as well. While this point is so obvious as to be hardly worth mentioning, the otherwise crucial exercise of determining the distinguishing features of medical ethics and "applied ethics" as a unique field of inquiry may have unintentionally obscured the issue. If these considerations hold up under further scrutiny, then careful attention to the three models described will be much more fruitful than they will be misleading for the beginning ethics instructor in the clinical setting. Furthermore, if the ethics instructor takes those models seriously the chances are very good that he will end up defining himself in one way or another as a change agent within the current setting of medical education and clinical training. The important difference will be that he will see himself as a change agent who has important allies already securely in place within this system, if he can but find them and apply the lessons to be learned from them to his own field of inquiry.

ACKNOWLEDGEMENTS

An earlier version of this paper was read before the Westminster Institute, University of Western Ontario, and I would like to thank the Institute staff for their helpful comments and criticisms. My colleagues in the Medical Humanities Program, Michigan State University, especially Tom Tomlinson, made useful suggestions for the final version.

ON BRIDGING THE THEORY/PRACTICE GAP
IN TRAINING MEDICAL ETHICISTS

Charles H. Reynolds, Ph.D.
John A. Eaddy, M.D.
Karen K. Swander, Ph.D.

Those vocations and professions that provide services that impinge directly on human flourishing are inevitably embroiled in an on-going debate that centers on the relationship of theory to practice. This is as true of medical ethics as of other vocations and professions.

The Problematic

In philosophical ethics and social theory, the theory/practice problematic frequently arises as an epistemological question; but that epistemological question will not be directly addressed here. Rather, we want to approach the theory/practice problematic in a somewhat different form. We will review how those of us who planned the clinical medical ethics graduate program at the University of Tennessee have wrestled with how best to prepare men and women to function in an informed and effective way as teachers, counselors, advocates, critics, decision-makers, researchers, and negotiators in medical ethics. Although different skills and competencies are required for these various medical ethics roles, one trait is central for each of them: a capacity for and training in discerning judgment i.e., we want to suggest how we have been instructed by our colleagues in other practice-oriented fields in this effort to develop discerning judgment in our students.

Our experience has shown that a philosophical resolution of the skeptic's questions about the adequacy of moral theory for guiding actual decisions is not required prior to planning and implementing a programmatic way of enhancing discerning judgment. We do not need to claim either a capacity to make perfect judgments ourselves or a solution to the epistemological puzzle about the relation of theory to practice in order to recognize that some judgments are more discerning than others.

Kai Nielsen has argued[1] that traditional approaches to applied ethics are in shambles because metaethics and normative ethics cannot provide the ideal theoretical foundations required for one to be an expert in applied ethics. His skeptical attack could be directed against any vocation or profession that provides services perceived to impinge directly on human flourishing. The skeptic serves as a reminder that human claims to knowledge about the theoretical requirements for human flourishing must remain provisional and in important respects are always pretentious and inadequate.

A Practical Response

But we must not allow the admitted strength of the skeptic's theoretical case to lead us to abandon the enterprise of enhancing discerning judgment. For non-ideal knowledge, which is the only knowledge that human beings can have, can be more or less adequate for enhancing human judgment.

That is Albert Jonsen's important point.[2] Jonsen has proposed that in his capacity as an educator of medical students and graduate physicians, he does casuistry on a daily basis and that he finds important resources and guidance in the casuistical tradition that enable him to do his work better and more effectively. We in the University of Tennessee Inter-Campus Graduate Program in Medical Ethics have discovered similar resources and guidance for enhancing discerning judgment by working closely with colleagues in other academic disciplines which include supervised clinical experiences as a central facet of their educational programs.

By framing the theory/practice problematic with reference to the skills and competencies that we believe our students should possess (and that are in that limited sense ideal aims), we share the perception of some of our colleagues in clinical and counseling psychology, medical education, legal clinical education, social work, and related fields; and, by approaching the issue in this way, we have discovered that the theory/practice issue is not as obtuse or as limited as one might otherwise be disposed to think.

Presuppositions of Clinical Supervision

A supervisor of clinical experiences can and should have an operational understanding of the theory/practice problematic, grounded in a notion of how to enhance discerning judgment, which he or she communicates to the student and uses in evaluating the student's performance. At one extreme, some supervisors communicate expectations and standards of discerning judgment to students merely implicitly by serving as role models, as well, perhaps, as by providing gentle reactions and suggestions to students in an indirect and supportive way. At the other extreme, some supervisors serve as a role model and also provide the students with a detailed listing of the skills and competencies required for discerning judgment, and then the students' performance is evaluated with reference to these explicit criteria. But at both of these extremes, and in the range between them, the supervisor both implicitly and explicitly communicates criteria and expectations for discerning judgment and evaluates the stu-

44

dents' actual performance in ways designed to enhance the development of discerning judgment. In short, specifiable skills and competencies provide the operational bridge between theory and practice in a supervised clinical education program. Supervised clinical practice as a mode of education is a means of assuring that the student has the necessary discerning judgment to make use of theory to inform practice before the supervisor will certify that the student has the knowledge and skills required for competent professional or vocational practice independent of supervision.

Medicine is the preeminent example of a profession using supervised clinical experience to enhance discerning judgment and in this way to bridge the theory/practice problematic. Clinical rounds with the physician-teacher as supervisor and role model are the **sine qua non** or medical education. The student's knowledge of the art and science of medicine--and, in particular, her/his skill in applying that knowledge to the case at hand--is continually evaluated and enhanced as he or she is supervised on clinical rounds while a medical student, and then later as he or she is provided increased responsibility under supervision as an intern and resident.

The knowledge and skills required for discerning judgment in diagnosis and treatment represent broadly shared aims of medical education. Even the national specialty examinations are calibrated to assess the discerning judgment of those who have been through the various supervised clinical experiences required as preparation for taking them. Indeed, at a highly abstract level, discerning judgment in diagnosis and treatment which bridges the theory/practice problematic can be seen as the ultimate goal of medical education. Theoretical knowledge is necessary but not sufficient for developing discerning judgment. Howard Brody[3] points out, in his description of the "good basic sciences instructor," the importance of reducing the theory component of early medical education to a manageable quantity of relevant material. But even when limited to those aspects of theory that are fairly directly relevant to clinical decisions, there is still a gap between the abstract knowledge of this theory and the application of it to the individual patient in practice. The skill of when and how to appropriate and use one's theoretical knowledge (and, in contrast, when to refer the patient to a specialist) is learned in, through, and by one's participation in supervised clinical experience. As a role model, the medical educator aims to empower the medical student to bridge the theory/practice problematic and to develop his or her capacity of discerning judgment in diagnosis and treatment.

But to empower their students to bridge this gap, medical educators must themselves stay abreast of the theoretical knowledge in their field. It is, therefore, critically important for

45

medical education that basic research be conducted in medical schools and teaching hospitals. Otherwise, the theory/practice gap could not be bridged adequately through the supervised clinical experiences in medical education due to paucity of theoretical in-put. Bridging theory and practice is an on-going and daily occurrence in medical education; it is intrinsic to the structure of the activity. There is no purely theoretical solution to the theory/practice problematic in medical education. There is only a social and structural solution. This solution is programmatic. When students are empowered to make discerning judgments in diagnosis and treatment, the programmatic solution has achieved its ideal aim. But physicians have not been made infallible or incapable of erroneous judgments. They remain subject to the human condition.

Although medicine provides a broadly-recognized model of a profession that bridges the theory/practice problematic by using the supervised clinical experience to enhance and evaluate discerning judgment, similar educational models are present on a more limited basis in law school legal clinics, in clinical and counseling psychology programs, and in other fields. We do not intend to explore these alternative clinical supervisory models in detail at this time. We do however want to suggest that in each of these instances the general aim of the supervised clinical experiences is the same -- to enhance the students' capacity to make discerning judgments as a way of bridging the theory/practice gap.

Furthermore, it is important to distinguish these types of supervisory clinical models from "real-world" experience models where the students are not under educational supervision while practicing the skills of a profession. Because of the anti-theoretical bias in our culture, these "real-world" experience models probably widen instead of bridge the theory/practice gap.

Clinical Supervision and Theoretical Pluralism

One might intuitively agree that supervised clinical practice facilitates bridging the theory/practice gap for physicians, psychologists, and lawyers, but nevertheless claim that this is feasible only because each has a broadly-shared theoretical knowedge base and that this feature distinguishes each of these fields from moral philosophy. This is not correct. There are important areas of theoretical agreement and disagreement in each of these fields.

In moral philosophy, for example, there is broad theoretical agreement on: (1) the philosophical constraints and characteristics associated with taking a moral point of view; (2) the general factors that lead to distortion in moral judgment; (3) a range of **prima facie** normative rules and principles that

46

apply to individuals and institutions; and (4) a range of questions that a complete theory of morality must address. Indeed, it is precisely this broadly-based theoretical agreement that permits Stanley Hauerwas[4] and Alasdair MacIntyre[5] to designate the "standard way" of doing moral philosophy as a focus for criticism. Nevertheless, there are important disagreements at the theoretical level of moral philosophy on the rational method of structuring and justifying a normative theory of ethics. Similarly, in medicine, there is wide agreement on what can be described as medicine's "scientific basis," but there is disagreement on whether the patient is the individual, the family unit, or the public at large, as well as on the treatment of choice for many types of cancer, heart disease, and brain dysfunction.

But these sorts of agreements and disagreements in theoretical orientations within a field of knowledge are not cause for alarm as long as the reasons for agreement and disagreement are continually investigated and debated. And that is happening in medicine, law, psychology, and moral philosophy. It is an educational travesty when students pursue a graduate program in any of these fields and do not learn alternative and even contradictory ways of conceptualizing and understanding the theoretical knowledge that is foundational for the field. Discerning judgment is required in selecting theoretical orientations as well as in applying theoretical knowledge to practical situations. The human condition does not lend itself to either finality or certainty in theoretical formulations of the knowledge base of any profession or field related to human flourishing. Our human judgments in this arena are at best comparative and discerning. And this is part of the reason why supervision in the clinical context is indispensable as a way of enhancing and evaluating a student's capacity to make discerning theoretical selections and to use theory wisely and skillfully when making practical decisions. That is why clinical supervision provides an excellent opportunity for bridging the theory/practice gap.

The irony is that moral philosophy—which has long been thought of as practical reasoning—would be so slow in coming to the realization that instruction in a practical setting is an excellent way of teaching, learning, and applying its own distinctive theory and skills. We can anticipate that, in due time, those who supervise clinical ethics students will make similar contributions to moral theory that clinical supervisors have made, for example, to psychological theory.

Clinical Practice in Medical Ethics

In the remainder of this chapter, we intend to describe the aims that we have for students in our Inter-Campus Graduate Program in Medical Ethics at the University of Tennessee and the ways that we use supervised clinical practice to realize these aims. Primarily, we intend to empower our students to make discerning moral judgments in their roles as philosophers with special competencies in medical ethics.

A medical ethics student is first of all a graduate student in philosophy. He or she must demonstrate similar competencies to other graduate students by passing a wide range of graduate level courses and preliminary field examinations.

In addition, medical ethics students take added courses in moral theory and a range of courses in medical ethics. Only then are students admitted to the supervised clinical courses in medical ethics; and only after completing background theory courses. It is these supervised clinical courses that represent the distinctive strength of the University of Tennessee program -- and the parallel to practical training in other fields.

Students entering the graduate program are first introduced to grand rounds and then to clinical rounds in a teaching hospital setting. After two years of limited clinical experiences, the students spend four months in an intensive and supervised clinical practicum at the UT Center for the Health Sciences in Memphis. After the students return to the Knoxville campus, they continue regular participation in supervised clinical rounds at the UT Memorial Research Center and Hospital. After their third year of study they enter a second intensive supervised practicum. Most students do this supervised practicum at the Lakeshore Mental Health Institute in Knoxville, although others return to Memphis and some choose an alternative setting. Every student must take two intensive supervised clinical practicums. By the time a student has passed all preliminary examinations and written a dissertation, he or she will have had extensive supervised experience in a clinical setting.

The Committee on Graduate Study in Medical Ethics that is primarily responsible for the medical ethics concentration is composed of seven philosophers, four physicians, one religious ethicist, one social scientist, and a chaplain from the Lakeshore Mental Health Institute. This committee meets on a regular basis to review and plan for the concentration, to screen students for admission, and to prepare and evaluate student examinations. Because the clinical practicum is an integral part of the medical ethics concentration, there has been no difficulty in having full participation from the physicians in all aspects of the committee's work. This participation of the physicians in the program has been critical to our success in obtaining and maintaining access to the teaching hospitals in Memphis and Knoxville for the supervised clinical rounds for the students. The chaplain from the mental health institute has been equally critical for maintaining access to that facility. Without this type of access and assistance from professionals with an established role in the

48

setting, a clinical program in medical ethics would not be a feasible undertaking. One cannot bridge the theory/practice gap adequately by the discussion of isolated cases and issues in a seminar setting. If cases and case discussions could be adequate in this regard, law schools which teach by the case method would certainly not go to the expense of establishing clinical education programs.

Some Basic Points

Once we describe the objectives for the students who participate in clinical rounds, it will be evident that to meet these objectives a medical ethics student must learn to bridge the theory/practice gap. We have learned from our colleagues in other clinical areas as we have experimented with different ways of empowering our students to bridge the theory/practice problematic. One important lesson we have learned is that supervisors must work with each individual student to assist that student to discover his or her own way of dealing with the theory/practice gap. Personality strengths and dispositions shape the distinctive way that each student resolves this issue. The solution must fit the student. Although some philosophical purists might find this admission troublesome, it is a solution that is present in medicine, psychology, and law, as well as in clinical ethics. Practitioners in these professions must also find a solution to the theory/practice issue that fits their distinctive personality strengths and dispositions. Professionals are also persons; it is not merely their clients who are persons. To conceptualize professionals merely as roles is just as inappropriate as to conceptualize clients merely as objects.

The critical importance of the personality strengths and dispositions of professionals for locating the proper solution of the theory/practice problematic for each individual practitioner is one reason that the theory/practice issue in medical ethics does not lend itself to a purely theoretical solution. Medical educators and supervisors of psychology students have long recognized the need for each of their students to discover his or her own distinctive way of bridging the theory/practice gap. In this respect, we have learned something of what it means for practical reason to be personal reasoning. Students have to "know themselves" before they can become competent medical ethicists. And supervisors have to know themselves and their students before they can become competent instructors in clinical medical ethics. Although students and supervisors must have a good knowledge of moral theory, an individual solution to the theory/practice problematic is not a logically derived solution. On the contrary, it is practical and personal. This recognition makes evaluation more difficult for the supervisor and the student. The student as a person is evaluated, not merely the student as a role performer. This is a difficult assignment for those of us who have long assured our students that we evaluated their work and not them. The supervisor does and must evaluate the student.

Objectives of Clinical Practice

The supervised practicums provide faculty in the program an opportunity to assist each student to resolve the theory/practice problematic in a way that fits his or her personal strengths. To assist the student in developing the discerning judgment that is the inclusive goal of all work in the clinical practicums, there are four general objectives that we have for the students and several distinctive skills that we expect them to learn. Supervision is our way of constantly reinforcing and assessing the student's progress in achieving these objectives and mastering these skills.

The first objective is that each student enter on a Socratic quest to know himself or herself and to understand himself or herself as a medical ethicist with a distinctive role in the clinical setting. Students are in the clinical setting to learn and they are not present as guests or as intruders. Their programmatic status entitles them to be present. It is nevertheless understandable that many of their associates who are also present for programmatic reasons (medical students, interns, residents, some of the medical faculty, etc.) in the clinical setting will not know why the medical ethics students are there. The student in medical ethics must develop the self-confidence to interpret his or her presence and role as a student to inquisitive associates. The student needs to be able to explain the importance of clinical experience to the development of the field, to communicate effectively with people who are suspicious of his or her "right" to be present in the setting, and to observe what is happening within (and how he or she relates to) the immediate clinical environment.

The student must develop a good self-understanding to relate effectively to others in a way that is conducive to learning in the clinical setting. It is for this reason that we gradually introduce the student to the clinical setting in ways that maximize the support from the supervisor. Furthermore, during the intensive practicum experiences, frequent small group discussions are conducted by the supervisor and private sessions with each student are regularly scheduled. These interactions assist the student to gain self-knowledge and self-confidence while undergoing what are frequently highly stressful experiences. As would be expected, some students learn that clinical medical ethics is not for them. Others become more deeply committed to this role directly as a result of their intensive clinical experiences. Our objective is that students gain a self-understanding of how and why they relate to this role as they do.

The second objective is that each student learn how to function in the role of an ethicist in the clinical setting. The role model of the supervisor is of critical significance if this objective is to be met. But it is also essential that the student have the background and training in ethical theory and in the literature of medical ethics if he or she is to know how to ask ethically significant questions and to observe ethically significant interactions and details. Students win respect from their medical associates in the clinical setting by being rigorous in their analysis of and comments on ethical issues, and by demonstrating a knowledge of the literature in medical ethics. As student become comfortable in their role as medical ethicists, they are often sought out and consulted by associates who initially were skeptical or critical of their presence. These informal consultations in the clinical setting are powerful reinforcements for the medical ethics students.

The third objective of the clinical experiences is that students gain a first-hand knowledge of the different institutional roles, of the administrative and authority structures, and of the institutional culture in several different health care and hospital settings. This objective is fostered by rotating students through a variety of institutional settings during their clinical experiences, and talking with them about the similarities and differences that they perceive in these settings, especially with reference to how patients and their families are treated. It is the responsibility of the supervisor to assist the student to gain a balanced perspective on these matters and to understand them as structural features of health care in this country. There is an initial tendency for students to be either apologetic for or critical of the medical and administrative personnel with whom they are working. But it is not our goal to train either apologists or critics of the health care system. We are comfortable with students who are either apologists or critics (or some of both) so long as they are informed about the matters they are addressing.

The fourth general objective is that students learn to identify the public policies that implicitly and explicitly shape and structure the different types of health care available to patients. The legal system, the system of third party payments, administrative regulations, professional licensure, national and state economic policies, and a range of additional considerations all affect how health care is structured and delivered. Although it is a challenge for any of us to view health care within a social policy context, one cannot understand the clinical practice of medicine without viewing health care in a broad societal frame of reference. Instead of clinical experience narrowing the students' perception of the social policy dimensions of health care, we have discovered that it helps them to recognize the importance of these broader issues. Courses in social philosophy

51

and legal medicine are frequently elected by students after they have been through an intensive practicum experience.

A student in clinical supervision develops a personal style of bridging the theory/practice gap as he or she makes progress in attaining these four general objectives and learns the skills to make discerning moral judgments.

Developing Discerning Judgment

We can now observe how clinical experiences aid a student in developing his or her skills in discerning moral judgment. As described in objective two above, the student must learn to function in the role of ethicist in the clinical setting. We are now concerned with how a student learns to function as a person who can make discerning moral judgments in the role as ethicist. Although this is a personal achievement for each individual student, there are nevertheless different moments in discerning moral judgment that we can isolate and describe. What is distinctive for each student is how he or she learns to relate these moments to bridge the theory/practice gap. It is the practical, synthetic moment of judgment that is distinctive for each medical ethicist, each psychologist, each physician, and each attorney. When this practical moment fits the personality strengths and dispositions of an individual, and reflects his or her theoretical understanding, it may be recognizable as a habit or style that is distinctive for that person. Creative judgment, although it may have an habitual pattern, is always involved in bridging the theory/practice gap. The creative moment in discerning moral judgment can be nurtured but cannot be directly taught. As mentioned above, professionals are also persons. Any proposal to bridge the theory/practice gap at the expense of what distinguishes human beings as individual persons must be rejected. But this rejection does not mean that we cannot describe different moments in discerning moral judgments. That we can and should do.

Consider the following example. You are in and out of a busy emergency room in a large hospital. You observe that an elderly woman has been sitting in the same chair over a three hour period. You see that she appears to be in pain and you know that the average waiting period this morning is approximately two hours. You go over and talk with her and it emerges that her son brought her in almost four hours earlier but that he did not register her and that she has not been able to register herself. You assist her in registering and ask the clerk if it would be possible for the woman to be seen immediately given her long period of waiting and her pain. The clerk politely informs you that she has to call patients in the order they have registered unless their condition requires immediate attention. The clerk asks you to assist the woman back to her chair and says that she

52

will be called in approximately two hours. How do you come to a judgment about what you should do in response to the clerk's comments?

The first moment in discerning moral judgment is to identify and describe the external factors to which you are responding. Are you bothered that the son did not register his mother? Are you concerned that no one else offered to assist her, or that you yourself were slow in responding to her plight? Are you upset by the rigid way the clerk follows procedures? Are you angry because the clerk refused your request? Are you confused as to why the woman did not request assistance from anyone? Do you feel that you have done your good deed by helping the woman register and making a request of the clerk so that now you can get on with more important matters? Do you feel a need to talk with the elderly woman to know how she is responding to the clerk's request? Before a discerning moral judgment can be made about what one should do in response to the clerk's request, we first need as full a description as possible about what the factors are in the situation to which we are reacting. You and I may immediately think that we should respond in very different ways because we are in fact reacting to significantly different descriptions of the same request. You may be reacting to the clerk's refusal to revise normal procedures while I am responding to her son's negligent behavior. Although we think we are reacting to the same event, we are in fact responding to two very different events. It is not unusual for moral disagreements to be rooted in different descriptions of what is perceived to be the same event.

As one way of addressing this issue, we recommend that our medical ethics students take social science courses that require them to develop the skills to observe and describe the verbal and non-verbal communications that occur in the health care setting. As students develop their observational and descriptive skills, they enhance their capacity to make discerning moral judgments. They are able to describe more completely what it is to which they are reacting. As their descriptive skills improve, the students are also able to communicate more effectively with their associates in the clinical setting.

The second moment in discerning moral judgment involves an ethical interpretation of the importance and nature of the event to which you are responding. Was the elderly woman treated unfairly even though regular procedures were followed? Was the clerk negligent by failing to observe that the elderly woman needed assistance? Was the registration desk staffed to operate effectively and efficiently? Was the son primarily responsible for his mother's plight? Did the woman not request help because she has been acculturated to be docile and patient? Would kindness require one to place the woman's name at the head of the registration list? If you interpret the event to which you are responding as an act of fair application of procedures (though perhaps an inadvertent wrong largely because of the son's neglect), and I interpret the same event as a denial of what elementary kindness requires, we may disagree in our moral discernment because we are applying different ethical principles to the event. If we discuss our disagreement, we may discover that we both believe that the woman was treated fairly but unkindly. We may also agree that the son was irresponsible in not registering his mother. As our students develop the skill to make discerning moral decisions, they become adept at providing good reasons to support their judgments.

Although anyone can appeal to an ethical principle to support a decision, a skill of selectivity is involved in discerning the particular ethical principle that is most appropriate for guiding a particular decision. Before we get to the point of arguing the importance of this or that particular principle, however, we need first to interpret to one another why you and I appear to select different principles for guiding our decision in a given situation. We may discover that the situation is more complicated than either of us had perceived, and then perhaps we can proceed to find a way to negotiate our disagreement. Or we might reach an impasse because you do not believe kindness is a relevant principle in the situation while I think it is the overriding principle. We may **understand** our **disagreement** even if we cannot reach agreement. Reasoned disagreements can occur over moral discernments just as they can occur in any other areas of judgment.

The third moment in moral discernment involves an anticipation of the response to our judgment or action. Let us assume that we both agree that the clerk was overly rigid in following regular procedures and that kindness would have led the clerk to place the elderly woman at the head of the registration list. Let us further assume that we both have a limited knowledge of the clerk's supervisor. You anticipate that a call to the supervisor would lead her to direct the clerk to place the woman at the top of the list. I anticipate that such a call would be futile because the supervisor would support the clerk. At that point, what would be a reasonable action for you would not be a reasonable action for me. And if we could not reach agreement about a prediction as to how the supervisor would be likely to respond, we would again have reached an impasse on how we should act in the situation. Anticipating the responses to our action or judgment is an important moment in moral discernment whether or not we believe that the morality of the action is determined by the consequences. In view of our different anticipations of how the supervisor will respond, you may decide to make a request to the supervisor and I may decide to lodge a formal complaint with the supervisor. But at that point we are taking two different actions because of our different anticipations of the supervisor's likely response.

Clinical supervisors are in a good position to assist students to develop this skill of anticipating the likely response to their judgment or action. This skill can be cultivated much better in a specific institutional setting than it can when we are discussing hypothetical cases. In an actual institutional setting, students do in fact get reactions to their judgments and actions. Sometimes the most critical reactions provide excellent opportunities for the supervisor to build instructional points upon.

Our anticipation also needs to address the policy issues related to this case. Are there, for example, policy changes that could be made in the registration process that would minimize the likelihood that this problem would be repeated? The moment of anticipation in discerning moral judgment is critical in assessing policy options.

The fourth moment in moral discernment involves a loyalty to the community of persons committed to reasonable moral judgments. It is the moment in which one anticipates the assessment of one's judgment or action by others who are also committed to enhancing moral community. It involves a readiness to be accountable. Regardless of how you or I would decide to act in the situation described in our case example, we should stand ready to be accountable for our judgment and action. Indeed, our action should be calculated to enhance the development of moral community. The supervisory relationship is ideal for helping students develop the skills associated with this moment. The supervisor, however, must be careful not to abuse this moment by elevating himself or herself to the position of a representative member of the moral community. This is perhaps the most difficult moment for the supervisor because as a member of the moral community the student is the supervisor's peer.

Conclusion

We had to make a choice between responding directly to Nielsen's skeptical diatribe against applied ethics or responding indirectly by suggesting a very different way of approaching the theory/practice problematic. Our position is that the theory/practice gap represents an opportunity for creativity and thus that it is not one more indication that philosophy and the human imagination are bankrupt. Nor do we need to look beyond the humanities to be rescued from a dire predicament into which we have been thrust because of the poverty of the western philosophical imagination. The quest for certainty in the human sciences is always elusive. But this is not an argument for skepticism or a reason for despair. Nor does it mean that the quest itself should or must be abandoned. It may be that the human imagination is such, and the human **proprium** such, that the quest for ethical certainty is fated to represent both the most admirable aspirations and the finite capabilities of homo sapiens.

Religious affections which locate the certainty in cosmogonic myths of world beginnings or eschatological myths of world endings have the virtue of being able to affirm that ethical certainty is both imaginable and beyond the reach of humans living after the beginning of time and before the end of time. Ethical certainty is associated with either the quest for the return to the ideal past or the quest for the entrance into the ideal future. An imaginative certainty is affirmed at the same time that the immediate realization of that certainty is denied. Those who need the solace of certainty to resolve the gap between theory and practice in medical or applied ethics can and should find solace in a religious cosmogonic eschatological myth.

Those who can accept the responsibility of creatively overcoming the theory/practice gap, however, while recognizing that every attempt to overcome it represents a risk and an adventure, may discover that their affections are oriented to a creative power shared by themselves and others that permits them to achieve satisfaction in the present without requiring either past or future certainty.

In its finer moments, even the casuistical tradition reviewed by Jonsen accepted responsibility for human creativity and abjured certainty as a human achievement. The casuists recognized certainty as a quest but recognized the probabilistic status of human judgments. They did not make the leap from the judgment that human certainty is impossible to the assertion that normative moral reasoning is bankrupt. Instead, they recognized that some reasons can be better than others even if certainty and perfection exceed human capabilities.

Although we have focused in this chapter on how moral discernment can be enhanced through a clinical medical ethics program, this can also be accomplished in the supervised learning environment of the college or university classroom. In that context we must assist the students to become active participants in a learning environment as we supervise and facilitate their learning. Although none of us can hope to accomplish as much in a single class as can be accomplished in a planned program of study for graduate students, any achievement in this respect is not to be dismissed lightly.

FOOTNOTES

[1] Kai Nielsen, "On Being Skeptical About Applied Ethics," this volume, pp. 93-113.

[2] Albert Jonsen, "On Being A Casuist," this volume, pp. 115-127.

[3] Howard Brody, "Teaching Clinical Ethics: Two Models for Consideration," this volume, pp. 31-42, especially pp. 36-37.

[4] Stanley Huerwas, **TRUTHFULNESS AND TRAGEDY** (Notre Dame: University of Notre Dame Press, 1977), especially Chapter One.

[5] Alasdair MacIntyre, **AFTER VIRTUE** (Notre Dame: University of Notre Dame Press, 1981).

THE MEDICAL ETHICIST AS AGENT FOR THE PATIENT

Robert M. Veatch

The topic for this exchange raises questions about what clinical medical ethics is, how it fits into therapeutic relationships, whether it violates or enhances them, and if it does enhance them, whether that is a good or a bad thing.

Thus, before addressing directly the topic of whether a clinical role for medical ethics violates or enhances the therapeutic relationship, we need to try to clarify what we mean by clinical medical ethics and what we mean by therapeutic relationships, as well.

First, then, what do we mean by clinical medical ethics? In the history of medical ethics, most medical ethics has not been clinical. Medical ethics is the analysis of the moral rightness or wrongness of actions in the medical sphere. Most of that analysis has taken place within religious traditions, in theological debates, in philosophy classrooms, in courts and legislatures, and in the mass media. In fact, it has often been argued that the only way we know what is right or wrong in a specific clinical situation is by absorbing some more general ethical stance, explicitly or implicitly, and applying it to a specific problem. Clinical medical ethics, then, is that relatively small part of medical ethics where we put our ethical stance to the test of an actual, concrete, decision involving a specific medical choice dealing with a single individual's health. We can only act, especially in a crisis, when years and years of preparation that is not specifically clinical prepares the way to on-the-firing-line concrete choices.

Moreover, most clinical medical ethical choices surely do not take place in a traditional relationship between a physician and a patient. Many occur in newer, more complex health care settings involving other health care professionals--nurses, emergency medical technicians, pharmacists, and so forth. The vast majority surely involve no medical professionals at all. Most certainly involve lay people acting alone or with other lay people. When a parent chooses to risk his child's welfare by not taking him to an emergency room for an asthmatic attack in order that he may continue devoting attention to other family needs, he makes a clinical ethical decision. So does a woman who chooses not to abort a pregnancy. When a priest advises that a parishioner's treatment is extraordinary, he makes a clinical ethical decision.

I take as the key feature of a clinical medical ethical choice that it involves a specific, live case problem faced by a

lay person or a health professional or both. It may arise within
a health care setting such as a hospital or a physician's office
or may be outside the traditional medical settings such as the
home, in a lawyer's office, a priest's confessional, or
elsewhere.

Someone trained in ethics may be involved in a number of
ways. Clinical teaching with interns, residents, faculty, and
health professional students may deal with specific cases, but
the ethicist may not actually interact with the patient whose
case is being discussed at all. Rarely does a day go by when
humanists working in medical ethics do not get involved directly
in cases. Some portion of that teaching and counseling involves
only the physician, nurse, or other health professional. In many
other cases they are involved directly with a patient or family
member having to make a critical medical ethical choice without
ever encountering other health professionals. Patients may come
to see them in their office; they may meet in neutral settings
such as a restaurant; in a minister's office; or, in a hotel room.
Only in rare circumstances does an ethicist interact with both
patient and health professional, and even then it is not always
in a hospital or some other health professional turf. Yet in all
of these cases, they are engaging in clinical medical ethics.
The focus shifts from the more general, historical,
philosophical, systematic thinking toward a specific live case
where someone has to make a decision affecting one individual
patient.

If the claim about the complexity of clinical medical ethics
is correct, then the answers to the questions raised in this
first exchange are going to be extremely complicated. For
example, it is asked whether the ethicist needs the permission of
the patient to be present at case discussion, consultation,
examination and treatment. But certainly if a patient calls at
the ethicist's office and asks to come to see him about a medical
ethical problem, any question of the patient's permission to be
present at the consultation is moot. Likewise, it is not exactly
the right question if the ethicist is asked by a physician to
help him sort through his options for some problem he faces.
Certainly there is a privacy question raised by any disclosure
between physician and ethicist, but it is not a question of being
in the patient's presence. That seems to be a question reserved
for that relatively small percentage of clinical medical ethical
encounters when both patient and health professional other than
the ethicist are present, usually in a hospital.

There is one final preliminary problem: is the medical
ethicist's role to be construed as an analytical one or one more
directly advocating certain medical ethical choices? Probably
the answer to the questions raised about violating and enhancing
the therapeutic relationship will depend upon which model is

chosen. Most ethicists are usually more comfortable with the analytical role. They help sort out the ethical options, the kinds of reasons that support various options, and the historical precedents for options from different religious and secular traditions. We cannot rule out, however, a role that includes giving direct advice or, in the extreme case, even making the decision for the patient. This might arise especially if the medical ethicist is working within the patient's tradition and the ethicist has been engaged specifically for the decision-making role. There is nothing wrong with the orthodox Jews engaging Rabbinically trained ethicists to do directive counseling or even actual decision making for certain kinds of cases.

The problem of whether the clinical medical ethicist is a neutral analyst, teacher or is more directive arises for other professionals. Lawyers, architects, accountants, public policy analysts, psychotherapists, nurses, and physicians all face the problem daily. It is striking that it is primarily health professionals who cling to the more directive, active decision-making role while most other professionals now acknowledge that expertise in a particular profession does not give one expertise on the values needed to make choices about how a professional's skills shall be used. An architect does not try to tell a client whether to build a Victorian or a contemporary home the way a physician still sometimes tries to tell a patient whether to have a radical or a simple mastectomy or whether to have by-pass surgery.

One other professional group often remains very directive in its teaching and counseling. That is the clergy. Even Protestant clergy, with their more egalitarian doctrine of the priesthood of all believers, do not shun the prophetic role; they speak forcefully and directly on some of the most controversial ethical matters facing their parishioners--matters as controversial as mastectomy and by-pass surgery. They advocate certain life-styles for their lay people and feel comfortable in that role.

There is a key, unique feature in the clerical role that may help us understand the conflict between neutral analysis and a more directive role for medical ethicists and physicians. The clergy have been chosen by lay people explicitly because they are expected to advocate, teach, prophesize, and counsel based on a set of beliefs and values that the lay person has affirmed. When--and only when--the lay person has explicitly affirmed a set of values shared by the professional--cleric, ethicist, or physician--is such a professional justified in taking up the more directive, value-affirming role. That virtually never happens with the physicians and only rarely happens with medical ethicists. It would happen if a physician were working within a

61

health care system that had a specific set of values endorsed by the patient--a physician at Oral Roberts Medical Center, for example. It would happen if an ethicist were working within such an explicit value-affirming health care setting or if the ethicist were engaged by the patient because of the value framework with which he is identified. I cannot imagine how this would ever happen if the ethicist were doing clinical medical ethics as a consultant to the professional, rather than the patient, except in rare cases where an entire health care system is value explicit.

This creates a real problem: it means that ethicists and physicians in the moral therapeutic setting of today ought to remain value-neutral, unless invited by the patient or by the public image of the institution to take on a more value-affirming role. The problem is that we now recognize that real value-neutrality is impossible for any person with professional expertise. It is impossible as a practical matter since all of us are influenced by our beliefs and values. More important, it is theoretically impossible since professionals must use values to make choices within their professional role: choices about how to organize information, what information is important enough to present, and when relations with clients should begin and end. This means that clinical medicine as we know it today--except for those rare instances where medicine exists within an explicit value framework--is inherently compromised. The value-neutral role is impossible, yet the patient has not endorsed the value system the professional must use. Physicians and medical ethicists **must** incorporate their value systems into their professional work even though those receiving their services have not asked for the system of values they are receiving. When medical ethicists consult, both physicians and patients necessarily get **some** value framework. The ethicist--in contrast with the physician--should have been trained to be able to describe that value system and to identify it when it necessarily creeps into his work; and it will creep in.

Having said this, it seems that the obvious role for the clinical medical ethicist is as an agent for the patient. The patient, or the lay agent for the patient, should be presumed to be the primary decision maker for his or her own case. This should especially be the case when the decision involves ethical or related value choices. If so, the various professionals involved in the patient's case should all be seen as agents accountable to the patient. This is true for physician, nurse, and no less for a clinical medical ethicist. The unique ethical mandate of all clinical relationships--whether physician, lawyer, or clinical ethicist--is the professional's promise of loyalty to the client. A covenant is established in which the professional promises to remain loyal to the patient, respect the autonomy of the patient, and serve the patient's welfare within certain limits. One of the most important limits is any limit on the professional's judgment placed by the patient whose integrity and dignity the professional must respect.

If a direct covenant with the patient is the ethical foundation of the clinical medical ethical role, most of the problems anticipated in the typical discussion of that role—including the questions raised in the program announcement for this session—seem to vanish. There is no longer any question whether the clinical medical ethicist (or anyone else) must have the permission of the patient to be involved. Of course he must, just as anyone else involved must.

One of the problems of the American Hospital Association's "Patient's Bill of Rights" is that this document, generated largely by professionals, at points appears to bestow on patients a part—and only a part—of the rights they already possess. For example, the second point of the Patient's Bill of Rights grants to patients the right to information necessary to participate in decisions about their own care. But then in the next paragraph it places a severe and morally indefensible limit on the right by saying that in cases where the patient would be harmed by disclosure of adequate information, that information should only be given to relatives. The provision not only violates the patient's legal and ethical right to the information, but also authorizes a violation of the confidentiality between physician and patient by permitting information about the patient to be transmitted to a third party without the patient's prior approval.

The provision of the Bill of Rights presently under discussion—the one specifying that those not directly involved in the patient's care must have the permission of the patient to be present, implies that such permission would not be needed for those who are involved in the patient's care. Certainly at least an implied permission of the patient is required whether or not those involved are providing direct care or not.

If, however, the clinical medical ethicist is an agent of the patient and the basis of the relationship is a covenant established between the patient and the ethicist, this becomes a non-issue. One cannot imagine how the covenant could be established without the patient giving an adequate permission for the ethicist to be present. That is true whether they meet in the ethicist's office, in a public place, in a hospital, or in the patient's home. (One can envision a debate over the question of why ethicists don't make house calls.)

Viewing the ethicist as an agent for the patient also solves the problem of whether the ethicist should strive to be as analytical and as neutral as possible or should counsel specific courses of action based on his or her own value framework. As part of the covenant between the patient and the clinical ethicist, there would have to be an understanding about what role the ethicist should play. If the ethicist is engaged to provide analysis, description of alternatives, historical survey of moves that have been made in various ethical traditions, etc., then that becomes the role. If, however, the ethicist is engaged because he stands in a particular system of beliefs and values, one shared by the patient, and the patient wants recommendations for ethical action based on the ethicist's personal ethical judgments, then such an arrangement can be specified in the original covenant binding them together.

Likewise, the problem of confidentiality becomes moot if the clinical ethicist is an agent for the patient. The patient discloses only those things he would want to disclose. If the ethicist is to see the patient's medical chart, the patient will authorize it. If the patient wants certain areas to remain private, he will so specify.

Of course, in some situations the patient is in no condition to be an active partner developing a covenantal relationship with an ethicist trying to assist the patient in making the critical ethical choices about his care. Some patients are infants or small children who cannot decide for themselves. Others are too sick or too senile to function as competent medical ethical decision makers. In such situation, however, some other lay agent appropriately steps into the decision-making role: parents do so routinely for small children; the next of kin or someone the patient has designated while competent appropriately becomes the lay agent for the patient for decisionmaking purposes. The lay person, in turn, may appropriately turn to others he or she trusts for guidance in helping with difficult choices. Often the person to whom the lay agent turns will be another family member, a clergy person, a close friend, or relative. Sometimes, however, the lay agent, just like the patient, may turn to a clinical medical ethicist for some kind of assistance. They may enter into a covenant just as the patient would with the ethicist.

It is clear that the ethicist is not always seen as accountable first and foremost to the patient. That is unfortunate, but, in some cases, may be necessary. In case conferences on the hospital floor, ethics rounds, and in many private consultations, the ethicist is forced into a position of dealing only with the health professional involved in the case. When this happens, two quite separate role relations may exist. The most plausible, most easily defended interchange between a clinical ethicist and some other health care professional would deal with a very special set of ethical problems. It would not deal with the question of what the physician or other health professional ought

to do to the patient--to turn off the respirator or do a radical
mastectomy. Those are fundamentally, irretrievably the patient's
choices and no ethicist should deal with anyone else in such a
way that the decision will be made for the patient without the
patient's full participation.

Occasionally, however, the health professional faces a
different kind of ethical problem. It is an ethical problem
posed for the professional growing out of a set of choices the
patient has made. How should an anti-abortion gynecologist
respond when his patient has decided in favor of an abortion?
How should the oncologist respond to the patient who insists on
Laetrile? What should the physician do who is asked by the local
state prison to participate in an execution using medical rather
than traditional means of execution? What should Howard Levy
have done when ordered to train Green Berets in a way that he
thinks will eventually lead to entrapping Vietnamese villages and
thus violate his conscience as a moral human being?

Professionals are moral agents just like patients. For
every set of choices a patient may make, the professional is
faced with a corresponding set of choices--about whether to
continue in the lay/professional relationship, about how to
determine his or her priorities, and about what to do when a
professionally articulated ethical stance conflicts with a
personally held one. In all of these cases the professional
becomes a primary moral decision maker who may turn to an
ethicist in just the way a patient might. As with the patient,
health care professionals might not choose to look to professional ethicists for either clarification of options or more
directive moral advice. Should they choose to do so, however,
they have the right to establish a covenantal relationship with
the ethicist just like the patient did. Physicians, nurses, or
other health professionals become temporarily lay persons seeking
professional services the way they might turn to a lawyer for
legal assistance or an accountant for accounting assistance.

The second way in which the physician may turn to the
ethicist for help is quite different. The physician may want to
present to his or her patient a set of plausible options for
dealing with the patient's problem. When those options involve
ethical dimensions, the physician may want to turn to the ethicist as a consultant to help sort out the alternatives and what
the ethical arguments are for and against various options. If
the physician chooses to do so, it is precisely analogous to the
times when that physician turns to a cardiologist to sort out the
treatment options for a patient with cardiac insufficiency or to
an oncologist to clarify options for the treatment of the cancer
patient. Here the ethicist becomes a consulting professional
brought into the margins of a patient's case for a specific
purpose.

Normally the physician presumes the permission of the patient for such formal or informal consultation unless the patient says otherwise. If a fee is involved, that permission probably should always be explicit, but when the physician turns to a colleague on a hospital staff for gratis counsel we normally assume no explicit patient permission is necessary. It is not obvious that this is the right answer. Maybe physicians should always disclose to whom they are turning for help in order to seek the patient's approval. If no information can be transmitted in a value-free manner, then maybe the patient should consent to the value messages the physician gets from the consultants. There is no reason to think that the requirement for patient permission should be any different when the consultant is a clinical medical ethicist rather than a clinical oncologist. Both groups of professionals have certain canons of objectivity toward which they strive (knowing they can never fully succeed). Both groups deal with highly controversial issues necessarily involving value judgments even when they try to limit themselves to matter-of-fact and "reasonable opinion." If explicit patient permission is required for one, it should be required for the other. If one group of consulting professionals is exempt, then the other should be as well. In the consulting role the clinical ethicist has exactly the same relation to the physician as any other clinical consultant.

Having explored how the clinical medical ethicist might be involved in various therapeutic relationships, we are still left with the question of whether that involvement violates or enhances the relationship. If this analysis is correct, we are dealing potentially with two separate, independent therapeutic relationships: one between patient and physician, nurse, dentist, or other traditional health professional; the other between the patient and the clinical ethicist. It is nonsense to ask whether the involvement of the clinical ethicist enhances the therapeutic relationship between the clinical ethicist and the patient. The therapeutic relationship between the patient and other health professionals, therefore, must be the one being addressed. Keep in mind that clinical ethicists can impinge on the relationship in several ways: acting in an independent covenantal relationship with the patient, acting directly with the health professional to deal with the professional's own ethical problems, caused by the patient's decisions, or, finally, as a consultant to the professional to assist in developing options to be presented to the patient.

In each of those therapeutic relationships the ethicist may well cause problems as well as enhance the relationship. If he does cause problems, however, it does not follow that he has necessarily **violated** the relationship. Suppose, for example, that a clinical ethicist working independently with Karen Quinlan's family suggests the option of having the parents force the physician involved in the case to stop a respirator. He might, as Father Trepasso did very responsibly in that particular case, inform the parents acting as agents for Karen, that the physician's insistence on continued respirator treatment is unacceptable in the tradition of Catholic moral theology of which the patient, the parents, and the priest are a part. There is no question that he seriously disrupted the therapeutic relationship and that we should be forever grateful to him for doing so. He acted as an independent clinical ethics consultant, in this case standing within the moral tradition of the patient and the lay agents for the patient. In doing so he helped destroy one therapeutic relationship and helped build another. In helping destroy the first, it should not be said that he violated it in any way. In building the other, he certainly improved the quality of the care the patient received. In the end the critical question is not whether the presence of the clinical ethicist enhances or harms the therapeutic relationship. It is whether the ethicist in a clinical role remains faithful as an agent of the patient, keeping the covenant that binds them to one another.

CLINICAL MEDICAL ETHICS AND THE LAW
RIGHTS AND DUTIES IN ETHICS CONSULTATIONS

John A. Robertson

A significant development in the last ten to fifteen years in the healthcare system has been the emergence of medical ethics as an integral part of medical education and medical care. Revelations of excesses in human experimentation, the emergence of life prolonging technologies, such as heart and kidney transplants, respirators, and dialysis, and the rising consumerism of the 1960's, made physicians and the public aware that much of medical practice involves non-medical ethical, legal and social questions beyond the expertise of medicine itself.

One response to this awareness has been exogenous regulation of medical decisions by publicly articulated legal rules and norms, such as the HHS rules for human experimentation, laws about brain death, informed consent and the like. Here the power and authority, indeed legitimacy of medical hegemony has been questioned and directly confronted by substituting public norms for the non-medical aspects of medical practice. The tension here is between public and professional control, with an ever shifting balance among these elements.

A second development has been endogenous incorporation into medical education and training of ethical training and awareness. The assumption is that if doctors face and make ethical decisions, then they should have training in such matters. This response has led to courses in ethics, law and related aspects of medical care in almost every medical school in the United States, and the employment of philosophers, theologians, lawyers and humanists by medical schools. It has also led, as part of this teaching role, to increasing involvement of philosophers, theologians and lawyers in clinical medicine, as consultants and advisors to physicians, through attendance at the bedside, during teaching rounds and on IRB's. A closely-related development has been the rise of in-house, hospital ethics committees that may be consulted by physicians on a mandatory or optional basis as ethical problems arise, usually in the care and treatment of critically ill and dying patients.

We see, in short, the development of a new clinical role -- an addition to the health care team that in some cases may be as important as the roles assigned to its medical members. While the reasons for the emergence of the role are understandable, its scope and institutional posture is less clear. The rights and duties of role occupants are also unclear. This paper will discuss the legal aspects of clinical medical ethics, or medical ethics consultants, looking first at the physician's right and duty to consult or utilize the services of an ethics consultant, and then turning to the legal rights and duties of the consultants. The goal is to produce a preliminary mapping in order to clarify and define institutional parameters of the ethics consultant.[1]

I. The Physician and the Medical Ethics Consultant

At the present time medical ethics consultants function largely as an adjunct or assistant to physicians, either as individual consultants, or as members of institutional committees which physicians choose to consult on an advisory basis. (On rare occasions individual patients or families may consult an ethicist for help with a medical care decision.) Though not invariably so, ethics consultants become clinically involved only with the members of institutional committees which physicians choose to consult on an advisory basis. (On rare occasions individual patients or families may consult an ethicist for help with a medical care decision.) Though not invariably so, ethics consultants become clinically involved only with the consent or request of the physician. This situation raises two issues: (1) the physician's legal right to call in a consultant; and (2) the physician's legal duty to do so.

A. Physician's Right To Use An Ethics Consultant

The question of a physician's right to use an ethics consultant concerns whether he is at liberty to do so, rather than whether he has a claim right on others to provide one.[2] The main issue here is whether consulting an ethicist or institutional ethics committee violates any legal or ethical duty the physician has to the patient. Two possible issues arise here. One involves the broad area of confidentiality and concerns whether the physician may discuss a patient's case with another without that person's consent. That is, must the physicians ask the patient's permission to seek an ethics consult? Must he inform him if he does?

The answer is probably not. Confidentiality is an important value in medicine, but it has never functioned to prevent physicians from seeking advice or consultation from others who may assist or improve the physician's handling of a particular case. Indeed, the patient is deemed to give implied consent to the physician seeking advice from others that are reasonably likely to help in management of the case. As Mark Siegler has recently shown,[3] as many as 75 people may in a case of routine surgery have legitimate access on the basis of implied consent as members of the total health care team to a patient's medical record. A physician who discusses a case with an ethicist or a hospital ethics committee would presumably be acting for the patient's best interests as part of the care of the patient and would be

70

privileged to do so as a matter of implied consent, unless the patient had given an explicit order to the contrary. Indeed, the law would not even require that the patient be informed that others have been consulted or had access to his records.

Bringing the consultant to the bedside is another matter. Here the relationship of the ethicist to the patient should be handled similarly to the handling of relations between other consultants and students in the presence of the patient. Whether we take partnership as the controlling image of the doctor-patient relation with the patient informed and cosenting to all transactions, or a more paternalistic physician-guided model, simple courtesy and respect require that any consultant be introduced to the patient or patient's family and remain only with their permission. If prevailing practice or custom, as is no doubt often the case, does not generally inform the patient about the use or presence of a consultant, there would appear to be no reasons why the ethicist should be treated differently. For the sake of consistency, the physician may be discourteous in either case.[4]

The question of a physician's right to resort to an ethics consultant presents an issue of the physician's discretion in management of a case. The patient's role in agreeing to or even being informed of the situation is secondary even though consent to procedures or decisions made as a result of the consultation may be required. The consultative nature of the relationship between ethicist and physician emphasizes the great respect for physician discretion in management of a case that the relationship entails. The physician is consulting an ethicist for advice, clarification and analysis of the ethical issues involved. He is not transferring decisional authority to him. As with other consultants, the ultimate decision about management of the case rests with the physician (and the patient), in light of the clarification and analysis of the consultant.

Given the consultancy arrangement, a physician would have no legal duty as such to take any particular action as a result of the ethics consultation. His obligation to the patient continues to be to possess and use that degree of skill and care possessed and used by reasonable physicians in the circumstances. While this duty may require seeking an ethics consultation and considering the advice proferred,[5] it requires the physician to act only as a reasonable physician would in light of the information received. Thus, unless the decision is removed totally from the physician, there is no duty to follow the ethicist's advice or recommendation, though there is a duty to act reasonably in light of it. An ethics consultation will prevent a physician from claiming ignorance of the moral gravity of a situation, but the consultation alone will not mandate that the physician take any particular action.

B. Duty to Obtain an Ethics Consultation

While the physician may be free to consult an ethicist without violating any duty to the patient, a major issue is whether the physician is ever under a duty to do so. Physicians use consultants all the time. A central principle of medical ethics is to seek a consultation when management of a case indicates the need. The law imposes this duty as well, and will award damages to patients who have been injured by a physician's failure to seek a consultation where other reasonable physicians would.

Does the physician's legal and ethical obligation to call in a consultant extend to an ethics consultant? There is a plausible case that it does in at least two circumstances.

The first, and least controversial, is that there is such a duty when the hospital or institution explicitly imposes it, as it does with research with human subjects and sometimes with termination of treatment of the critically ill. In that case, failing to refer a case to an IRB or other ethics committee would violate an institutional, and in some cases, a state-imposed rule, and could lead to damages on the basis of a negligence per se rule.

At the present time, with the exception of human subject committees (IRB's) most institutions do not require ethics review or consultation. A survey by the President's Commission for the Study of Ethical Problems in Medicine found that only 17 hospitals of more than 200 beds in a sample of 400 had ethics committees, with seven of these in New Jersey, where you would expect such committees to have been formed as a result of the guidelines formulated in the Quinlan case.

A major issue about the use of ethics consultants thus concerns the extent to which hospitals and institutions should institute and create ethics committees, and then require that they be used in certain cases. This issue actually depends on a preliminary judgment that ethics committees are needed to prevent erroneous or inappropriate decisions in certain cases. Questions to be addressed concern defining the category of cases which warrant review; designing a review process that will enhance accuracy without undue cost; deciding whether review should be mandatory or optional and, in either case, whether the ethics committee's conclusion is merely advisory or must be followed by the physician. While ethics committees are not now well-developed or widely used other than in human experimentation, there is currently widespread interest in them and likely to be further development and expansion of their use in the near future. Although a complete discussion of them and their impact on the moral issues that arise in medicine are beyond the scope of this paper, their role and function as a type of collective or group ethics consultation on a mandatory basis should be noted.

More controversial is the question of a duty to seek an ethics consultation when no hospital or institutional rule specifically requires it. The question of such a duty would arise, of course, only if an ethics committee or consultant were available on the premises. A legal duty to seek an ethics consult would exist if a physician could be ordered to pay damages to a patient for failure to have obtained an ethics consult. The question thus is one of negligence: is it professional malpractice not to seek an ethics consult in certain cases? To find a doctor liable for not seeking an ethics consult and thus the subject of a legal duty to do so would depend on (1) the difference or impact an ethics consultant could make in the handling of the case, and (2) the custom or practice of other physicians or the reasonableness of calling for an ethical consult.

Under existing principles of malpractice law, damages could be awarded for not seeking an ethics consultation only if the consultation would have improved the handling of a case. It seems clear that an ethicist or ethics committee could improve the handling of a case in many situations. While a physician may have had some college or medical school exposure to ethical issues, physicians will not always be adept at seeing the ethical issues and problems that may exist. The extent to which issues of autonomy, beneficence and justice arise in a case may not always be obvious, much less how conflicts among them should be sorted out. Consider for a moment the complex ethical issues that arise in such typical cases as whether an elderly woman with a gangrenous leg may refuse amputation, whether parental wishes against surgery for a newborn with Down's Syndrome should be followed, or whether intravenous feeding for a comatose patient can be stopped.

It is not arrogant to think that consultation with an ethicist or ethics committee may improve a physician's decision in these cases, if only in clarifying the issues and conflicts, and making the physician aware of ethical, legal, and policy materials on such decisions. In many cases the consultation could lead the physician to make decisions that are more respectful of patients' rights or interests than he would without the consultation, for example, by showing how the Down's Syndrome child has rights to treatment that should be given priority over the parents' wishes, or that intravenous feeling may legally and ethically be stopped as the family wishes, even though the physician on his own would have continued them.

But though resort to an ethics consult could help patients, there would be no legal duty to do so unless the applicable standard of care for patients in those circumstances would require the consult. Under malpractice law physicians are liable for omissions only if reasonable physicians in the same or similar circumstances would have performed the action. Even if an ethics consultation would have prevented a decision detrimental to the patient, resulting from the physician's failure to consider an important ethical issue, a plaintiff would also have to show that other reasonable physicians in those circumstances would have sought a consultation. This standard depends in large part on the custom and practice of physicians. If a majority of physicians in those circumstances would recognize that there were non-medical ethical issues beyond their competence and seek an ethics consult, the case would be much stronger that there was a duty to consult (although the respectable minority rule would still provide a defense in many jurisdictions).

But a majority of physicians do not now seek ethical consults, and so no custom to that effect exists. However, it may still be possible to show or establish that a reasonable physician in those circumstances would call for a consult, and not act on his own. With all the attention given to medical ethics and the increasing intervention of public or societal norms into medical practice, a reasonable physician should now know that in certain areas, e.g., defective newborns, fetuses, the comatose, refusal of treatment, experimentation, etc., there are ethical issues beyond the physician's expertise concerning whether the public and law may have standards, and which should therefore not be decided by the physician without, at the very least, checking with in-house specialists on the subject.

A court holding that a physician has a duty to seek an ethics consult, even though not yet a custom among a majority of physicians, would be setting a standard beyond medical practice. While such decisions by courts usually engender protest and controversy about unjustified and inexpert interference with the practice of medicine (see, e.g., reactions to **Helling v. Carey** and **Canterbury v. Spence**), the question is whether such a requirement can be justified in its own right. It is unlikely that a court will so rule, but it is possible and there is no reason why they should not. Requiring a physician who is making a decision that will cause someone's death to reflect on it with an expert on the ethics and propriety of doing so seems a reasonable policy.

A further problem with maintaining a successful malpractice suit against a physician for failure to consult an ethicist concerns whether such a suit would lie in its own right, or whether it would bolster a suit on other grounds. That is, in most cases the suit will claim that the physician was negligent in handling the case for some reason beyond his failure to seek an ethics consult. However, making a decision on an ethical matter without expert advice could be evidence of negligence or recklessness. A physician who turned off a respirator or stopped feeding would be liable because it violated a duty to the patient, whether he had consulted an ethicist or not. If he defended by claiming that he had acted reasonably in good faith, he would have a harder time sustaining that defense if he had failed to consult an ethicist in a situation where reasonable physicians would recognize that a serious ethical problem existed.

II. The Legal Duties of the Ethics Consultant

A. Individual Ethicist

1. The Right to Give Ethical Advice: Licensing

Doctors, nurses, lawyers and other professionals must be licensed to practice their professions. Ethics consultants give advice and make recommendations that can affect the lives of doctors and patients in significant ways. Must they be licensed as well? At the present time, the medical licensing acts do not cover the kinds of advice and services that medical ethicists perform. A common definition of the practice of medicine is "suggesting, recommending, prescribing or administering any form of treatment, operation or healing for the intended palliation, relief or cure of any physical or mental disease, ailment, injury, condition or defect of any person...." While an ethics consultant could attempt to practice medicine, if he is truly being a consultant (e.g., in Terrence Ackerman's terms, "facilitating moral inquiry"), then even in recommending a course of action he would not be practicing medicine within the meaning of the medical practice acts.[7] Whether ethics consultants should be licensed in their own right will depend on future developments in the field and is beyond the scope of this paper.[8]

2. The Duty to Give Competent Advice

No cases involving ethics consultants have arisen, so the following comments about legal duties are based on analogies or generalizations about the legal duties that persons, particularly professionals, have when they undertake to perform certain tasks. Although malpractice suits against ethicists are so unlikely as to appear fancified, it is still useful to see what legal duties could apply in order to define better the obligations of the ethics consultant role.

The ethics consultant, like any other actor who undertakes to act, advise or provide services which could affect the lives or well-being of others in significant ways, could be held legally responsible for a failure to use due care and act reasonably in the consultant role. Such a question could arise in a suit brought by a patient or physician who claimed to have been injured by the ethics consultant's actions.

To win such a suit the physician or patient would have to establish (1) that an ethics consultant had a duty to meet certain standards in his advice, (2) that the consultant failed to do so, and (3) that the failure caused the plaintiff's injury. Let us examine each of these elements further.

A main issue would be to establish the ethics consultant's standard of care. As with physicians, the duty of care would depend upon what other reasonable ethicists in those circumstances would do, which would in turn be a function of the precise facts and situation. At a minimum the ethicist would have to have a reasonable level of competency in describing, clarifying and facilitating ethical analysis of a case, and then not overstep the bounds of analysis and clarification into normative ethics or substantive decision-making in its own right. In short, the duty is to be a good, competent, reasonably humble ethicist. The malpractice would be in poorly performing in that role, e.g., omitting or misinforming about a key ethical issue so that a major aspect of the case is missed, or preempting the decision by telling the physician what to do.

After establishing that the ethicist deviated in some significant way from good ethics or consultant practice in the circumstances, the plaintiff would then have to establish that the dereliction caused an injury. In the suit by a patient or patient's family, the claim would be that the ethicist gave or failed to give advice which led to a patient, for example, being maintained several extra days on a respirator, or that fluids were improperly withdrawn. In a suit by a physician, the doctor would have to show that as a result of the ethicist's advice he had been injured, and not merely that he had made an unwise or unethical choice. The clearest cause of injury would be if the doctor made a decision based on the ethicist's advice that led to criminal or civil action or disciplinary action against the doctor, and hence damages. In either case, theoretically damages would lie against the ethicist, though suits are highly unlikely, if only because the damages may not be large enough to support a tort action. Indeed, the most likely suit against an ethicist would arise if the patient were suing the doctor and hospital, and added other parties and consultants and defendants including the ethicist.

The theoretic possibility of suit does show the need for ethicists to use due care in their advice, and not to overstep their bounds (as well as to arrange for insurance coverage by the institution). Ethicists can give bad or wrong advice, just as any consultant can. They can be arrogant, as if they think they know what the correct answer is and insist that it be followed, or believe that they have an ethical duty to achieve certain goals, and thus arrogate to themselves certain decisions. While such types may be rare, and may not last long as ethics consultants, we must remember that ethicists too may act improperly.

To take but one example of consultant negligence (though not one arising in a clinical setting), consider the role that a priest consultant played in the Phillip Becker case, in which parents opposed treatment of a twelve-year-old Down's Syndrome child for a ventriculo-septal defect and were upheld by the courts. Most commentary has been critical of the parents' decision and the court result, because Phillip appeared likely to benefit, and his parents did not appear to be acting for his best interests. It turns out that the parents took the position that they did in part because of the advice received from a priest whom they had consulted about this case. It is not known whether the priest was trained in medical ethics, or what his reasoning was. At the hearing before the court, the Beckers stated that their consultation with the priest led them to their position of being firmly against treatment which the doctors thought would extend the life and prevent suffering in their retarded son. A more accurate ethics analysis might have led to the opposite result. While a suit against the consultant in this case may not have been appropriate, since causation would be difficult to prove, one can imagine similar situations where a physician relies on an ethicist and makes decisions that result in harm to the patient and the physician.

III. The Ethics Consultant as Whistleblower

Perhaps the most difficult issue in determining the ethicist's duties arises in a situation where the ethicist knows that a patient has been wronged. As Ackeman cogently shows, the main function of the ethics consultant is "facilitating independent moral investigation by health professionals."[9] It is not to be a moral policeman, who identifies instances of clearly immoral behavior by health professionals; a patient advocate whose prime duty is to protect the interests of patients; or a secular clergyperson whose duty is to inspire people to engage in morally appropriate behavior.

While this account of the ethicist's role is analytically sound, the question remains of what the ethicist consultant should do (1) if he thinks a morally inappropriate course of action is taken in a case on which he has consulted or (2) in other cases of which he is aware. Indeed, this issue is one ethicists are familiar with, because the question of duty to report wrong, or whistleblowing, by members of the health-care team is a common situation that ethicists discuss in their teaching.

The ethicist, of course, is in a similar bind. At some point he will have a duty to report, and even risk his job for it. Two situations need to be distinguished. One involves concern about institutional practices, and the other relates to questions regarding the care of particular patients.

A. Duty to the Patient

The issue here is whether an ethics consultant who is called in by a doctor in a particular case for consultation has a duty to protect the patient when he learns that the doctor, despite the consultation, chooses a course of action that, in the ethicist's view, harms the patient.[10] To take the repair of duodenal atresia in an otherwise health Down's Syndrome child as an example -- what should the ethicist do qua ethics consultant if the doctor, after hearing the ethicist's analysis of the child's rights, chooses to accept the parent's refusal of operative permission and orders that the child not be nourished.

The issue here is whether the ethicist, because of his involvement as consultant, takes on a duty to act for the well-being of the patient that did not exist before the consultancy, or whether his duty is merely to give a competent ethical analysis that will facilitate the physician's process of moral inquiry? If the ethicist's role is simply to facilitate moral inquiry, it would seem that he then takes on no independent duty to protect the patient. In considering this question, we are at the very heart of the ethics of consultation. The medical consultant is chosen by the physician, reports only to him, does not manage the case himself, and merely facilitates the physician's medical management of the case. Although I do not know of any cases on this issue, my sense is that the courts would find that the consultant would, if aware of the improper management that would clearly harm the patient, have a duty to protect the patient. By agreeing to advise the physician about this case, he takes on a duty to act for the patient's best interests. This duty includes rendering reasonably competent advice as a consultant, and arguably, acting in other ways to protect the patient when he becomes aware of them. Of course, the evidence of harm and need for intervention would have to be clear and strong for this additional duty. But in such cases, I think the courts would recognize it.

If the medical consultant has such a duty, then it is difficult to see how the ethics consultant should be treated differently. Although his role is to facilitate the physician's moral inquiry to help the physician and other decision-makers make appropriate decisions, he performs this role to help fulfill the goals of the doctor-patient therapeutic relationship, which includes some measure of respect and concern for the interests of the patient. As a matter of both ethics and law, it seems to me

78

that entering into a consultant relationship involves the assumption of a duty to act to protect the patient when aware of a clear threat of a significant harm. The scope of this duty and when it arises requires analysis of precise factual situations. But it seems to me that an ethics consultant who did nothing when the doctor acquiesced in the parents' decision could be found as civilly and criminally liable for not fulfilling a duty to the child as could any other member of the medical team.

B. Duties to Other Patients: Whistleblowing in the Institution

Here there is no particular patient about whose care the ethicist is being consulted. Rather, he hears or learns about an ethically dubious institutional prctice that affects some other patient or patients. Does his position as ethicist create a duty to act to protect other patients by calling unethical practices to the attention of the relevant actors, or reporting such practices to appropriate institutional or other authorities? Unlike the situation of consulting with a physician about a particular case, I do not believe that the ethicist has an ethical or legal duty to monitor, report, or otherwise improve institutional ethical practices to any greater extent than anyone else aware of them.

An ethicist may be more ethically sensitive and hence more likely to identify unethical conduct or practices than other persons. His greater knowledge may also increase his anguish, as he has to struggle more often and intensely about what to do about unethical situations. It may even be appropriate for an institution (or institutional committee, such as an IRB) to look to the ethicist to identify and bring to the attention of institutional authorities unethical practices, just as it might expect an institutional lawyer to raise legal problems that he sees. The role here would not be a moral policeman so much as ethics consultant to the institutional authorities, to help them design and run an ethically sound institution. But his role as house ethicist does not in itself create any greater duty to take action. A patient injured by an unethical institutional or physician practice of which the ethicist was aware and did nothng would have a much weaker claim that the ethicist's reluctance to act or speak out made him legally culpable for his injury.

If this analysis is correct, then the ethicist has no greater legal duty of whistleblowing than others. Such duties may, of course, arise as a moral or legal matter for all persons aware of an unethical situation. Imposing a higher duty on the ethicist would not be justified by his expertise in ethical matters. It might also place a barrier in the way of acceptance and resort to the ethicist by those who most need his services.

FOOTNOTES

[1]The issues here are really a subset of the issues that arise regarding the moral and legal aspects of medical consultation, with special differences arising from the non-medical nature of the ethics consultation. There is a long history of discussion in the medical literature concerning moral norms and rules of etiquette involved in the consultant role, having roots to some extent in the concern to prevent the stealing of patients. But the law is not particularly well-developed here. Consent and malpractice principles are simply applied to this new area.

[2]A physician, however, could argue that a well-equipped institution should have an ethics consultant available just as it does medical specialists and allied services essential to provide good care.

[3]Mark Siegler, "Confidentiality: A Decrepit Concept," **NEW ENGLAND JOURNAL OF MEDICINE**, 307 (December 1982), pp. 1518-1521.

[4]An ethicist aware that a physician has not followed such common courtesy will face a personal and professional moral dilemma about introducing himself to the patient or suggesting a different practice to the physician. This raises a variation on the whistleblowing issue which frequently will confront clinical ethicists, and which is treated further below.

[5]Indeed, since the role of the ethics consultant will usually be to clarify and describe, rather than to recommend or decide -- that is to do descriptive or metaethics rather than normative ethics, a recommendation may overstep the ethicist's rightful role.

[6]See, e.g., Ark. Stat. Ann. S72-604(1).

[7]Terrence Ackerman, "The Role of the Ethics Consultant: A Theoretical Analysis," unpublished manuscript. See also Ackerman, this volume, pp. 143-175.

[8]A question of whether ethics consultants practice law may also arise, since they often discuss cases, and indeed, may be the only available source of legal information to the doctor involved. Non-lawyer consultants should be wary of assuming that they know the law and can expertly advise physicians of it -- there have been too many mistakes of this sort.

[9]Ackerman, op. cit.

[10]The ethicist on the ethics committee may also face a dilemma of whistleblowing in a case about which his committee has been consulted. However, as one of a collective of consultants his duty is different than when he is a consultant to a physician in a particular case.

LEGITIMATE AND ILLEGITIMATE ROLES FOR THE MEDICAL ETHICIST

David C. Thomasma

Our interest in this section is to explore the ways in which medical ethics, as an applied venture, might enhance or detract from the role of the physician. In the papers from the other sections of the conference, opponents and proponents of the whole enterprise of applied medical ethics are represented. The questions we posed for this section, however, were aimed at our main object of the conference—assessing the impact of clinical medical ethics. Contributions to this section were asked to address the following specific issues:

Does a clinical role for medical ethics violate or enhance therapeutic relationships? The American Hospital Association's "Patient's Bill of Rights" states: "Those not directly involved in [the patient's] care must have permission of the patient to be present" for the examination and treatment. Could a medical ethics consultant be construed as one who is "directly involved in" care? Alternatively, is the function of the medical ethicist so remote from care that it would be inappropriate even to ask the patient for permission to have him/her present? Is there really a need for a medical ethics professional to be at the bedside? If so, what is the basis of this need; and does it outweigh the cost in terms of invasion of patient privacy and intrusion into the physician-patient relationship?

Although Professor Kai Nielsen, among others, raises the skeptic's question regarding whether there can be such a thing as medical ethics at all, Robertson and Veatch were not asked to address that question or formulate a response to it. Now that the conference has ended, it seems important to me to sketch what I consider legitimate and illegitimate roles of the medical ethicist from our experience. This sketch can function as a general description of roles of medical ethics in the clinical setting. At the same time that the description is offered, I intend it to be a partial answer to Nielsen's skepticism that it can be done at all. It has been done. It can be done. Whether or not it is being done properly or well is a genuinely philosophical question and is also partially answered in my remarks. However, I purposely avoided anticipating the positions and responses of later papers in the volume, lest too much be revealed at the outset. Nonetheless, I do comment on Robertson and Veatch in the final section of my presentation.

My comments on the role of the ethicist are entirely devoted to that of the medical ethicist, with specific reference to that role in the medical school and in the clinical setting of a teaching hospital. I am not sure to what extent these roles, for the role is actually plural, are capable of extrapolation to other situations. The reason for my uncertainty is that the roles are context driven, that is, derived from the peculiar nature of medical education, the goals of medicine, and the needs of ill persons.[1]

With that disclaimer in hand, however, I am sure of at least one thing--there are legitimate roles the ethicist can play. Precisely because the legitimate roles are the more difficult to accomplish and demand more than traditional academic behaviors (even demeanor), the illegitimate roles are more tempting. Not infrequently, they are forced on us by unsuspecting allies. Accordingly, my comments are structured as follows. First, I delineate what I consider illegitimate roles. Then I discuss those that are legitimate. Finally, I try to establish the criteria upon which my choices are based, since the latter will certainly appear arguable to some. In this section, I will also comment on the opinions of Robertson and Veatch.

One more note before I start. My comments are based on nine years experience developing two clinically oriented medical ethics programs, training four faculty, fifteen philosophy doctoral candidates, and over fifteen post-doctoral fellows in the hospital setting. Of itself, this experience does not ensure the validity of my remarks. It merely delineates the "population" from which they arise.

Illegitimate Roles

One could construct a litany of illegitimate roles. Out of this litany, however, I will pick six. They are: institutional ethicist; humanities validator; crusader of truth; resident moral expert; reformer; God squad. Let me start with the **least** innocuous.

1) Institutional Ethicist. The institutional ethicist role takes two forms. The first is "being called upon;" the second is political validation. "Being called upon" is analogous to a clergyman's role at a banquet, when he or she is asked to give the benediction. Placed in a medical school, the ethicist is often asked to ethically baptize, as it were, some policy decision, say a faculty wage hike schedule, or the structure of a student counseling service. Political validation of the institution is usually introduced by the remarks: "Now that we have an ethicist on board...," or "We are already doing ethics. We have X on board here...." Both roles are vacuous because objectives have not as yet been met; both are tempting because it seems that somebody is finally paying attention to ethics!

2) Humanities Validator. This is a dangerous role. The ethicist is cast or casts oneself as a legitimator of human sensi-

tivity, actually best left to those trained in the behavioral
sciences. Or the ethicist sees his or her role as confirming the
wisdom locked in all treatises of twenty centuries of "higher
thought." We all like to be portrayed as sensitive to human
beings, but ethics, as such, does not qualify us for this recognition. Besides it is a misperception of the humanities.[2] The
"higher thought" form of this role is equally pernicious because
the task in medical school is to validate medicine as a humanistic discipline, not to use patient care problems as ciphers of
past truth. Application of that wisdom, not confirmation, is the
authentic objective. Besides, as Max Black tellingly points out,
the entire humane studies educational program has to be re-
thought in our technological age because of its frankly elitist
purpose in the past.[3]

3) Crusader of Truth. One of the most frequently heard
stereotypes of ethicists is that they are more interested in the
truth than in care of the patient. This stereotype was posed
recently by William Ruddick.[4] To accept the role of crusader of
truth is to artificially claim that the medical professionaliza-
tion process is to be aimed entirely at patient care,[5] to the
exclusion of a search for truth. It also rests on a faulty metaphysics, that is, that truth, goodness, and beauty may not meet
transcendentally in the one. The search for truth in medical
ethics must be intimately linked with care for the patient
because medicine is defined by the medical relationship with
patients.[6]

4) Resident Moral Expert. This is an extremely problematic
role, often confused with the question about whether an ethicist
should make recommendations. It therefore should be carefully
distinguished from making recommendations. In fact, the moral
expert role is a pretentious posturing, because it rests on the
assumption, as Peter Singer classically describes it, that one
has the only true moral perspective, or that the study of ethics
eo ipso makes one ethical.[7] On the other hand, it is not
inappropriate for an ethicist to make recommendations for a
course of action,[8] recognizing the demands for clinical closure
in medical decision-making and that neither medicine nor ethics
is an exact science.[9] Because the ethicist in the clinical
setting is asked for opinions, it is easy for him or her to posture as a moral expert. It can be avoided by a dose of humility
and an awareness of the human condition in which we can only do
our best with decisions that must be made.

5) Reformer. Because the way medicine is taught and practiced sometimes does not live up to its ideals, many ethicists in
my experience have adopted the mantle of a reformer of the medical system, a sort of Ivan Illich prophetic role, without his
catholicity of learning.[10] Such an accusatory role fails on
several counts. First, one's training in ethics does not qualify

one to run a hospital, or a national crusade against medicine. Second, it is counter-productive to the legitimate recommendation role described above because its shrillness is amplified by physician sensitivities to criticism. Third, the fact that the ethicist is a guest of the profession is lost sight of. The partnership I have described elsewhere collapses.[11] Fourth, and most convincingly, the serious and demanding work in one's own discipline, which is after all a discipline of reason, is abandoned in favor of more emotionally satisfying fingerpointing.

6) God Squad. The "God Squad" role is the most pernicious of all. In it, the ethicist absorbs the roles of patient advocate and spiritual minister to the sick in an orgy of emotion. Without the barriers, and barriers they are, which protect health professionals in the midst of much tragic, human suffering, the ethicist lets his or her heart rule the mind. Frequent and unnecessary visits with the patient occur. Without proper training, the ethicist sometimes oversteps the bounds, offers advice to patients, becomes their advocate against some real or imagined assault on their dignity. At the core of this role is a failure to recognize the degree to which a sick person is an impaired person[12] and a failure to recognize the legitimate training of trained professional patient advocates and ministers.

Legitimate Roles

Having detailed six illegitimate roles, I now turn to describe eight legitimate ones.

1) Listening. Presence in the clinical setting allows us to listen to clinicians express their ethical concerns about a case as they develop. There is usually a cathartic moment after which initial reservations of the clinician are overcome, and after which he or she begins to develop a professional bond with the ethicist, encouraging the latter to consider a number of further problems for joint exploration. Many clinicians have explicitly stated that they prefer this bond to consultations with chaplains or the social scientists. But this may only be a matter of taste and intellectual stimulation.

2) Intuition Analyzer. I find that intuitions about the right course of action in a case are often expressed. These are analyzed and critically examined, usually after the catharsis mentioned in (1). The result of such analysis is greater awareness of the role of feelings, character, and professional style on the part of the physician as these roles enter clinical judgment. These are further separated from the ethical judgment in the case so that they may not be misconstrued as moral rules.

3) Reconciler of Accounts of a Case. Incredibly, I find that the ethicist, as an arm of the managing physician, often has

a clearer picture of a difficult case than many of the players in it, the patient, the housestaff, the nurses, and so on. Much of our time is spent pursuing leads, analyzing intuitions, and tracing third party statements ("The student said that the nurse said that the patient was uncooperative..."). This function occurs because we are usually called for consultation on a difficult case which, at the very least, involves clashes in values and corresponding complex emotional content.

4) Sketcher of Ethical Landscape. After the first three activities are accomplished to some extent, the ethicist begins to sketch the ethical landscape. It is not appropriate at this point to insist on one or another ethical theory. This function can best be understood as an initial description of the ethical parameters of a case. Without sufficient clinical experiences, ethicists often neglect the medical and institutional data important for this sketch.

5) Isolator of the Major Ethical Issues. This function establishes the ethical import of a case. It usually occurs when those involved are able to state that the case is one of consent, or autonomy, or the doctor's duty, or some other classification which aids in the discussion by eliminating extraneous issues. Often, at this stage, the ethicist will distinguish the ethical issues from those which are legal or economic. In a number of cases I find that health professionals think they are involved in a dispute about care rather than in a moral dilemma; for example, a question about whether IVs are to be considered ordinary or extraordinary means for a dying patient is sometimes perceived as a clash of care strategies and argued on that basis alone.[13] In examples like these, health professionals become surprised and even relieved to learn that the dilemma has ethical conditions. Perhaps their relief stems from the fact that they have exhausted all arguments about strategies for care and can turn to new considerations ethical reflections might have to offer.

6) Identifying and Ranking Values. Assisting those involved in the case usually involves a struggle to wrestle with all the conflicting values. Here the ethicist can greatly aid the professionals who often lack the skills to sort out and rank these values. "Which should come first: The patient request or my duty?" "The state law says that I have to have cessation of total brain function, but it seems inhumane to keep him alive when others need his bed." These statements suggest important professional, personal, legal and ethical duties. How are they to be ranked? If the decision is made without some explicit ranking of the values, I call it a knee-jerk decision, most often colored by emotions or the last person with whom one talked. Ranking requires ethical dialogue. It also requires the next step.

7) Provider of a Theory of Ranking. Reasons are given in the sixth function for ranking certain values above others, and so reaching a decision. These reasons are actually statements of ethical principle which for personal and professional reasons should bear some consistent stamp over the course of the years. The theory of ranking an ethicist can contribute, then, directly bears on decisions to be made by the managing physician. I find that if all the other functions have been properly carried out, this theory of moral weight to be given to conflicting values most often reflects a joint decision in the case, or at least reflects an ethically justifiable claim by the physician for his or her decision.

8) Making Policy Recommendations. Certain problems occur frequently enough to warrant the development of hospital or institutional policy. Resuscitation guidelines are just one example. These policies do not eliminate the moral reasoning process just described for each individual case.[14] But they do attempt to develop general guidelines, like those protecting human subjects in research, which help clinicians map the moral territory of a case more quickly, because some of the reasons in (6) and the theory in (7) have been discussed ahead of time. It is, after all, the mark of educated persons to anticipate future moral quandaries from their past experience. I find this function is more often fulfilled in joint research undertaken by the ethicist with clinicians, perhaps because the ethicist is disposed to the realm of generalization rather than particulars.

Criteria

It is only fair that I conclude with the criteria upon which I made judgments regarding illegitimate and legitimate roles. They are sprinkled throughout my comments and are presented here without the complete philosophical and theological justifications they demand. Comments on Robertson and Veatch are included.

1) Medicine is a relationship between doctor and patient. With Pellegrino I have argued that medicine is neither a science nor an art in the traditional understanding of those terms, but a theory about practice in this relationship.[15] Whatever the merits of the view that medicine is a relationship, the moral character of medicine must be seen as arising from the relationship and not as an externally imposed ethical system layered on to a value-free science.

Both Robertson, with his legal training, and Veatch, with his celebrated libertarianism,[16] view the matter quite differently. In their view, the ethical quandaries develop more from a clash between the patient's individual autonomy, recognized in normal life, and medical paternalism, which reigns supreme in the clinical relationship.[17] Put another way, the moral problems in

medicine are analogous to the moral problems in social ethics or
legal cases. They do not derive from any particularly unique
character of medicine. This point has bearing on differing
philosophies of medicine. It also has bearings on the assumptions about the proper role of the medical ethicist spelled out
in my paper.

Because Veatch and Robertson apparently see medical ethics
as a branch of social ethics or social policy, they do not consider that the ethicist in any way "disrupts" the clinical relationship. In their view, the consultative capacity provided by
an ethicist to patients is largely patient generated. It is not
seen as a function of the relationship between doctor and
patient, as I have described it. This difference of opinion has
strategic and educational ramifications noted in more detail
below.

2) Ethical analysis of decisions made in the medical relationship is an inherent, second-order function of medicine. In
other words, if the moral character of medicine arises from its
own **praxis**, then the obligation to reflect on its moral quandaries follows. Ethics is thereby not a "foreign" discipline
applied to medicine, but a reflective function of medicine
itself.

As might be anticipated from their positions explained so
far, neither Robertson nor Veatch would agree with this description. The importance of correctly describing the nature of medicine in a philosophy of medicine is thereby revealed. For it is
such a philosophy of medicine that underpins one's stance on the
function of the medical ethicist. Veatch's position, for example, derives directly from his work on covenants in medicine and
ethics. Both Robertson and Veatch immediately and explicitly
assume that medical ethics is a branch of applied ethics. The
rest of their respective positions follows logically from this
assumption.

Both assume that moral norms in medicine can be deduced from
general moral principles, a point I consider quite problematic.[18]
Although I agree that a medical ethicist may offer consultative
advice, he or she should do so both out of respect for traditional ethical systems as well as the values of patients, physicians, hospitals, society, and religious or cultural traditions
(the latter as emphasized by Veatch). The trick is not to function as an agent of any one of these views, but as an agent of
resolution within the relationship between physician and patient
itself.

In this respect, Nielsen's criticism of Veatch and Robertson
is especially damaging. If medical ethics is merely an application to medicine of applied ethics, then all of the traditional

questions of the skeptic about the legitimacy of applied ethics must be answered. If, however, some additional normative impetus for the resolution of cases can be provided by the aims of medicine itself,[19],[20] as MacIntyre suggests is possible for "practices" (cooperative human projects with their own standards of excellence),[21] then some answer to the skeptic's cautionary questions may be possible.

3) The ethicist brings to the second-order analysis in medicine noted in (2) certain skills and language the doctor and patient may not have, but is nevertheless a guest of the profession. Some colleagues have objected to my characterization of the medical ethicist in a medical school as a guest of the profession, on the grounds that medicine is fortunate to have the skills and insights of a humanities professional to underscore its humane tradition.

With respect to this point, Veatch does detail the way in which an ethicist might function as a consultant to physicians, but this is presented almost as an afterthought. The idea he emphasizes is that the best model for the medical ethicist is that of a patient advocate. Aside from the difficulties and confusions with standard patient advocates and chaplains his position causes, he has the role of the ethicist in the hospital completely reversed. The ethicist, as I have described him or her, is most often paid by a medical school.[22] This person is primarily an **educational** consultant. Presence in the clinical setting is seen as a prerequisite for proper training of medical students and faculty, in conjunction with the role model faculty, in the ethical resolution of patient care quandaries involving a moral dimension. Rarely, if ever, is the ethicist called upon to act as an advocate for the patient, though this role is conceivable. Hence, the fact remains that, unlike many other professions, medicine has cautiously welcomed the ethicist into its own curriculum. Until we have proved our insights and teaching are indispensable, some measure of diplomacy is required.

4) The skills and language brought to medicine do not certify the ethicist as an expert in moral judgment, nor do they qualify him or her for other professional roles.

I find most objectionable the notion, expressed by Veatch and Robertson, that the ethicist ought to act as a kind of patient advocate. The image one conjures up is that of a minister of secular humanism, who might have a kind of pseudo-chaplain role to persons otherwise not represented by any faith tradition. In this view, the ethicist would represent for the patient, I guess against the hospital or the doctors (as Veatch's examples bear out), the sunny traditions of liberalism, utilitarianism or deontologism as applied to the patient's own situation. The reason I find the notion objectionable is that it is a false picture of the realities of modern medicine. Patients rarely know what we do or what we are, much less ask for advice about their own humanistic traditions. If they do know, they usually raise their fist in a Marxist salute of solidarity with us and, in an unsophisticated way, urge us to keep on trucking, to really teach those doctors ethics, "because they need it."

Of course, a lengthy or more sophisticated discussion might take place, as it does in difficult cases, but here the stereotypes of adversarial relations between doctor, patient and ethicist, found in Robertson and Veatch, breaks down. My experience, by contrast, reveals an existential awareness that all of us are locked together in a morally challenging and tragic situation. A great deal of love and compassion are expressed during the discussions. They are rarely, if ever in my experience, dependent upon an adversarial model of the ethicist as patient advocate.

This is not to say that an adversarial basis does not occur from time to time. It does. When it does, the case goes to court. When that happens, the case becomes a matter of public debate, policy, and notoriety. Unfortunately, those ethicists and lawyers with little or no clinical experience often take these cases as models for applied ethics, rather than the more intimate, discretionary ethics that occurs 90% of the time in the clinical setting.[23]

5) The most effective role of the ethicist is that of a consultant who makes recommendations based on the literature and discipline of medicine, ethics and medical ethics. Indeed, the greatest danger which would impede this role is that, in a desire to get educational turf or to be so diplomatic as to be harmless, the ethicist might lose objectivity. In this loss, he or she might be tempted to become a physician advocate precisely because some physicians have relied on them as colleagues and friends. Protection of objectivity can be accomplished by a formal recognition of the consultant role.

6) Ethical considerations constitute only one factor among the many considerations the physician and patient must make in coming to a decision. Others are the nature of the disease, professional standards, clinical style, the patient's and hospital's social context, psychological factors and economic constraints.[24] The rich variety of those factors is rarely accessible to those applied ethicists who lack clinical experience. As a consequence, their writings, while valuable and philosophically interesting, rarely reveal the necessary ingredients of realism for clinicians.[25] Because of this lack, they are often condemned to discuss cases with one another, having little or no impact on medical education, hospital policy, or clinical decisions. This criticism does not apply to Robertson and Veatch,

whose thinking has led many physicians and ethicists to reassess their own positions.

7) Finally, although Veatch would urge us in a quasi-religious direction, tenure in medical schools is rarely awarded to prophets! The task of medical ethics is not ministerial, but intellectual within a context of compassion.

FOOTNOTES

[1]David Thomasma and Edmund Pellegrino, "Philosophy of Medicine as Source for Medical Ethics," **Metamedicine** 2(1981), pp. 5-11.

[2]Jurrit Bergsma and David Thomasma, "The Contribution of Ethics and Psychology to Medicine," unpublished manuscript.

[3]Max Black, "Some Tasks for 'The Humanities'," in **The Sciences, The Humanities and The Technological Threat**, Ed. W. R. Niblet, (London: University of London Press, 1975), p. 5.

[4]William Ruddick, "Can Doctors and Philosophers Work Together?" **Hastings Center Report** 11(April, 1981), pp. 12-18.

[5]Mark Siegler, "Cautionary Advice for Humanists," **Hastings Center Report** 11(April, 1981), pp. 19-20.

[6]Edmund Pellegrino and David Thomasma, **A Philosophical Basis of Medical Practice** (New York: Oxford University Press, 1981), pp. 170-191.

[7]Peter Singer, "Moral Experts," **Analysis** 32 (1972), pp. 115-117.

[8]Terrence F. Ackerman, "What Bioethics Should Be," **Journal of Medicine and Philosophy** 5(1980), pp. 260-275.

[9]Alasdair MacIntyre, "A Crisis in Moral Philosophy: Why Is the Search for the Foundations of Ethics So Frustrating?" in **Knowing and Valuing: The Search for Common Roots**, Ed. H. Tristram Englehardt, Jr. and Daniel Callahan (Hastings-on-Hudson, New York: The Hastings Center, 1980), pp. 18-35.

[10]Ivan Illich, **Medical Nemesis** (New York: Pantheon, 1975).

[11]David Thomasma, "Medical Ethics Training: A Clinical Partnership," **Journal of Medical Education** 54(1979), pp. 897-99.

[12]Jurrit Bergsma and David Thomasma, **Health Care: Its Psychosocial Dimensions** (Pittsburgh: Duquesne University Press, 1982).

[13]D. Thomasma, K, Micetich and P. Steinecker, "Are IV Fluids Morally Required for Dying Patients?" **Archives of Internal Medicine**, 143 (May 1983), pp. 975-978.

[14]David Thomasma, "Decision to Use the Respirator: Moral Policy," **Bioethics Quarterly** 2(Winter, 1980), pp. 229-236.

[15]Pellegrino and Thomasma, **A Philosophical Basis**, Chaps. 2, 5, and 6.

[16]Robert Veatch, **A Theory of Medical Ethics** (New York: Basic Books, 1981).

[17]David Thomasma, "Beyond Medical Paternalism and Patient Autonomy: A Model of Physician's Conscience for Doctor-Patient Relationship," **Annals of Internal Medicine**, forthcoming.

[18]David Thomasma, "The Possibility of a Normative Medical Ethics," **Journal of Medicine and Philosophy** 5(1980), pp. 249-260.

[19]Thomasma and Pellegrino, "Philosophy of Medicine as Source for Medical Ethics," <u>loc</u>. <u>cit</u>.

[20]David Thomasma and Edmund Pellegrino, "Toward an Axiology for Medicine," **Metamedicine** 2(1981), pp. 331-342.

[21]Adasdair MacIntyre, **After Virtue** (Notre Dame, Ind.: University of Notre Dame Press, 1981).

[22]Thomas McElhinney and Edmund Pellegrino, eds., **Human Values Teaching Programs for Health Professionals** (Ardmore, Penn.: Whitmore Publishing Co., 1981).

[23]Stephen Toulmin, "The Tyranny of Principles," **Hastings Center Report** 11(Dec., 1981), pp. 31-39.

[24]Albert Jonsen, Mark Siegler and William Winsdale, **Clinical Ethics** (New York: Macmillan, 1982).

[25]David Thomasma, "Medical Ethics: A Clinical Base," **Linacre Quarterly** 49(1982), pp. 266-276.

ON BEING SKEPTICAL ABOUT APPLIED ETHICS

Kai Nielsen

> Socrates' interlocutors have not found their lives, because they have failed to examine them. Wittgenstein's have lost their lives through thinking too much or in the wrong way.
>
> Stanley Cavell

> It has been a long time since we philosophy professors have had much of a share in helping the intelligensia as a whole see things as a whole.
>
> Richard Rorty

I

I have for the most of my more or less adult life been fiddling around with something like ethical theory. Yet, I choke on the term "ethicist" and I would not be caught dead making a claim to moral expertise. And I don't think I would start claiming it if I got better at what I am doing. I hope I am a tolerably reflective chap but I don't know right from wrong any better or, for that matter, any worse than a tolerably reflective check-out clerk. I -- or at least some of my peers -- have some expertise in analyzing moral concepts, in specifying the structure of moral argument and in laying out in a more or less nifty manner moral arguments (say a case for or against abortion). Some of us also have a kind of expertise about the history of ethics. We can come to understand and explain Aristotle, Kant or Sidgwick very well indeed. We can know what they said and why they said it; we can know something of the historical and social placement of their thought and we can become adept at comparing and contrasting these historical figures. We might--though we tend not to--even come to have the kind of expertise that would enable us to do for the history of ethical thought and for morality itself something similar to what Arnold Hauser's social history of art did for art.

There are, as well, more distinctively philosophical things we could and sometimes do develop in our repertoire. We might become adept at tracing out the implications of (say) rule-utilitarianism for some medical practice and we might become good at testing the validity of the arguments employed by moral philosophers. Indeed, we might even become adept at recasting their arguments, when need be, in various ways so as to render them

95

valid or at least not so plainly invalid. Still, these things would not add up to a knowledge of right and wrong.

We could call these various activities "moral expertise" or "the ethical expertise of the ethicist," if we so desired, but all that would be rather misleading. There is physics and applied physics, mathematics and applied mathematics, music theory and composition, architectural theory and the workaday world of architects. Each has its own tolerably clear domain of expertise and there are reasonably clear links between the more theoretical activity and the more applied activity. But this doesn't work out so well when we think about ethics. And this obtains whether or not we are assuming an engineering model or some other model in conceptualizing the relation between theoretical ethics and applied ethics.[1]

There is, or at least can be, expertise about what used to be called metaethics and there is expertise about the history of moral thought, but it is unclear what the links are between those activities and attempts to say what is right or wrong, good or bad in any kind of systematic or even not so systematic way. There was at least relief from boredom when roughly twenty years ago analytic moral philosophers came to the conclusion that they needn't be just rather bad philosophers of language ("applied philosophers of language" if you will) but could do normative ethics again. But the liberation has not paid off very well. Systematic normative ethical theory is not in a very healthy state. There has in the past decade been a lot of it, some of it clearly in certain ways impressive, but it is neither clear what it comes to nor what its links are with the construction of a critical ethics, practical moralizing or social advocacy or with what some like to call "applied ethics," or "practical ethics." Moreover, there has not been a clear facing of the critique of the very possibility of a normative moral theory given by such penetrating and diverse philosophers as Edward Westermarck, Axel Hagerstrom and John Anderson.[2]

It is not clear what, if anything, could count as a foundation for morality, moral truth (true fundamental moral propositions) or a **systematic** knowledge of good and evil. It is not clear that there is, or can be, anything substantial in normative ethical theory comparable to what it is possible to have in music theory or architectural theory (to say nothing of physics or biology) which would provide us with **such** a knowledge of good and evil.

II

Much of the extant systematic normative ethical thinking is on the Kant-Mill-Sidgwick axis. Leaning toward the (broadly) Kantian extreme, Alan Gewirth tries to establish a categorical prescriptivity which is rooted in a knowledge of the generic features of action.[3] Freedom and well-being are two things, Gewirth claims, that any rational being will necessarily want and will recognize as necessary for the fulfillment of his or her purposes. Now, if x is a rational being, she will recognize that and this statement (itself alleged to be a necessary truth) entails, Gewirth argues, the further allegedly necessary truths a) that she must claim the right to freedom and well-being, and b) that others are bound to act in accordance with those rights-claims. But such a high **a priori** road will no more work for Gewirth than it did for Kant. Even if a rational agent (someone able to make correct deductive and inductive inferences and who is appraised of the relevant empirical facts) must recognize that freedom and well-being are necessary goods, she does not **contradict** herself if she refuses to acknowledge that she, or anyone else, has a rights-claim on those goods or that anyone is **obligated** not to interfere with her having them or seeking them. She might not have such deontic concepts or (more plausibly) she might not choose to reason in accordance with such deontic concepts while still having the teleological ones. Recall that Gewirth is trying to establish entailments here and a fundamental norm with categorical prescriptivity that any rational agent (in the above astringent sense of "rational agent") would find it self-contradictory to deny.

John Rawls account is not in the above sense Kantian.[4] He would not try to establish substantive norms which it is self-contradictory to deny, but he too tries, or tried, to give us a systematic normative ethical theory. (Or at least that is a very natural way to read him.) But again, as the extensive and often careful criticisms of his work have made clear, Rawls has not shown why it is, or even that it is, that rational agents, with or without a rudimentary sense of fairness, must in the original position adopt his principles of justice.[5]

Alasdair MacIntyre is not on the Kant-Mill-Sidgwick axis. Like Richard Rorty and Stanley Cavell, he thinks that this standard way of doing moral philosophy rests on a mistake. Indeed, he is quite dismissive of such an approach.[6] It is, in his view, a fundamentally misconceived way of being philosophical about morality. In some ways he wants to go back to a rather historicized Aristotle.[7] But it is not clear that he wants to construct anything like a normative ethical theory. Perhaps a better way of putting it is that he does not think that in our cultural situation there is much point in doing anything like that. His way of approaching his subject matter is the mirror opposite of Gewirth's extreme ethical rationalism. But it is also very different from Rawls' approach or from the rather more standard approaches to moral philosophy that have grown out of what was once called the analytic tradition.

MacIntyre proceeds very differently than do most philosophers who work out of the latter tradition. There is, particularly in his most recent work, relatively little in the way of conceptual analysis or argument. Instead, MacIntyre makes a very distinctive use of the history of moral thought (indeed it is a broadly conceived history of moral thought). He takes quite different figures from that thought, often brilliantly juxtaposed and/or perceptively aligned, and places them clearly in the changing social contexts in which they wrote. (He uses the term in a rather extended way.) Even if he is right--even if that whole cluster of approaches as different as Hume's, Bentham's, Sidgwick's and Rawls' do end in a bog--it is not clear that MacIntyre himself has not, in as unequivocal a way, painted himself into a corner. Following Aristotle, MacIntyre claims that there is a human **telos** which gives us the basis for a coherent account of the moral virtues that is not relativistic. His account, for all its awareness of history and cultural context, is still an account which purports in its own way to give us an Archimedian point to critique practices and institutions. It will, that is, give us a critical moral vantage point which will enable us in some important way to transcend the perspectives of certain cultures, including our own. We can ascertain what human goodness is by ascertaining what fulfills the human **telos**. But it appears at least that such a conception presupposes an Aristotelian "anthropology," and perhaps even a cosmology, in which it could be said that man, **qua** man, has a distinctive function, purpose or essence, such that we could say, with some definiteness, what human beings are for.

We can in some reasonable way make judgments about characteristic human needs but even that, in various ways, is more tricky and more problematical than it is sometimes realized.[8] A sign--if indeed we had it--that we might be on the road to success here would come in the specifying, in some reasonably non-tendentious way, of what the **essential** needs of humans are and of what, in the achievement of human flourishing, their respective weights should be, such that, when need conflicts with need, and the various contending needs cannot be satisfied or cannot be fully satisfied, we would know, or could make a reasonable guess at, what priority to give to what needs. But it is far from evident that we have such knowledge. MacIntyre's own development (in earlier works) of the idea of essentially contested concepts should make him more sensitive to difficulties concerning such knowledge-claims than he now at least appears to be.[9]

If, alternatively, we stop talking about the function of man and seek to discover what is good by discovering what people characteristically seek, we have in effect returned to a very simple, and very vulnerable, form of the very Enlightenment project that MacIntyre has already firmly rejected.

Talk of practices (cooperative human activities with their own standards of excellence) will not help here. It is one thing to find out what a good farmer, flute-player, insurance-salesman, teacher or chiropractor is or even what a good parent, friend or comrade is and it is another thing again, though indeed a related thing, to find out what a good man is or what the good for man is.[10] As Wittgenstein has made us aware, both over time and over cultural space, there are these diverse, often incommensurate practices in human life with at least no apparent non-arbitrary ordering of them in such a way that we can know how it is that we should live or what sort of persons we should strive to be. It is not evident how, given MacIntyre's approach, there could be such an ordering. Perhaps a use of John Rawls' or Norman Daniels' method of wide reflective equilibrium would give us some way to approach the task of making such an ordering. But MacIntyre utterly rejects that methodology and he also appears at least to reject the full-fledged Aristotelian appeal to some concept of the function of man. But without it, and just sticking with his talk of practices, it is unclear how he can give us anything of any greater objectivity than he thinks he finds in the Enlightenment project and with it—that is, with a full Aristotelianism—he has a crusty old metaphysical doctrine with well-known difficulties which it would be very difficult to imagine MacIntyre defending.

The goods internal to all practices may themselves require the virtues of justice, courage and honesty. But the comparative weight given to these different virtues will vary and what they will come to with different peoples and in different practices will also vary. MacIntyre has no more given us an Archimedian point than have the various philosophers defending various forms of what he calls the Enlightenment Project.[11]

MacIntyre, as is characteristic of him, is self-conscious about this. He remarks that unless there actually "is a telos which transcends the limited goods of practices by constituting the good of a whole human life," we cannot attain the Archimedian point that has been the dream of non-skeptical philosophers. But MacIntyre has not shown us what it is, except in mythology or ideology, to conceive of human life as a unity such that "a certain subversive arbitrariness" will not "invade the moral life" and undermine our capacity to specify adequately a table of virtues. He rightly sees Nietzsche as his arch foe. But it is evident here that he has not refuted him. If we could say what a human being is and must be to be fully human, we could perhaps give such a rationale for or of the virtues. But we do not even know whether such an essentialist question makes sense.

III

Perhaps others can do better what Gewirth, Rawls and MacIntyre have failed to accomplish. Still, we have a long history of trying and failing to do this and we have in Gewirth, Rawls and MacIntyre three distinguished and very different contemporary attempts to construct a moral theory which would afford us systematic moral knowledge. If, as I have claimed, they fail to deliver, that is not an insignificant discovery. Moreover, we have the sustained, and in important ways rather different, classical attempts by Westermarck, Hagerstrom and Anderson, and in our very most recent history, by Monro, Mackie and Harman, to show that in trying to construct such a normative ethic we are trying to do something that is impossible to do.[12] I am not persuaded that their skeptical case is conclusive, but it is, particularly when taken in conjunction with the failure of recent attempts to construct such a normative ethic, a challenge not just to be shrugged off. Generally, I do not expect that getting a conclusive case is the sort of thing we should expect from philosophy or, for that matter, from any other non-mathematical intellectual discipline, but it seems to me at least that the case of the skeptical critic against objectivist theories is rather strong.[13] It certainly should give anyone rather severe doubts that we have available to us a firmly articulated normative ethical theory that affords us a systematic knowledge of good and evil, right and wrong, such that it could give ethicists confidence that they have a moral expertise that will enable them to chart the way in applied ethics.

The applied ethicist might try to get along with middle level bridging moral principles and remain agnostic about the competing normative ethical theories. But the escape appears at least to be an impossible one, for these general normative theories still seem to be there in various ways as background assumptions in work in biomedical ethics and other forms of applied ethics. Moreover, depending on which background assumptions are made, different middle level bridging principles will be appealed to and those which are commonly appealed to will be given a different weight, placement and elaboration depending on which ethical theories are lingering in the background. And sometimes incompatible theories are yoked together as part of an applied ethicist's assumed background beliefs. Without the assumption of any background theories at all, we would appear at least to have a mishmash of bridging principles that afford little rational guidance.

We might very well get along with meta-ethics being in shambles, but if normative ethics is as vulnerable as I have portrayed it, how can applied ethicists in any determinate domain claim knowledge of good and evil or, more troublesomely and appropriately, I believe, a knowledge of good and evil which is not also available to any reflective person without any normative ethical theory? Without even the latter, the ethicist can hardly reasonably claim moral expertise or ethical expertise. But without some theory-dependent expertise what is he? Indeed, how can we even speak here of expertise? But without some sort of expertise in ethics how can the ethicist reasonably expect in any applied context to give any advice or make any suggestions with any authority at all? Perhaps he knows something about medicine or clinical psychology and using that knowledge he can in certain circumstances give some advice that would have an important moral upshot. But there still is no **moral** expertise or **moral** authority involved here. Moral expertise looks very much like a Holmesless Watson.

IV

Is not the upshot of this, it might be responded, just a replay of ethical skepticism or indeed perhaps something worse: ethical nihilism or cynicism? And do we not know well-enough the pitfalls and paradoxes of such views and do they not wildly run against our most deeply embedded considered judgments and our sense of the moral life? I would like to block these "inferences."

What is needed here is clarification and elucidation and the drawing of some distinctions. I am taking very seriously a kind of ethical skepticism but it is a skepticism about **whole normative ethical theories**, including middle level theories of applied ethics. It is a skepticism about whether we have, or are likely to come to have, a **systematic** knowledge of good and evil. But such a skepticism does not entail that we can never know or reasonably believe that anything is right or wrong, good or bad.

I would like to **deploy** in the domain of morality an argument similar to the one that G. E. Moore once used against skeptics in epistemological or metaphysical contexts. Moore pointed out (in effect) that in a rather large cluster of standard contexts I could be more confident that I have two hands and that I put on my underwear before I put on my pants than I could be of any philosophical theory, no matter how cogently reasoned, that concluded that there is no external world or that time is unreal. It is more reasonable to believe the empirical truisms and assume that somewhere there is a yet undetected **lacuna** in the philosophical argument than to accept the philosophical argument and reject the empirical truisms.

Similarly, in moral domains, it is more reasonable to believe that we know or can reasonably believe or reasonably securely accept that it is wrong to kill people just for the fun of it, torture the innocent, treat a person simply as a means to

101

one's own ends, routinely fail to keep one's promises, break faith with people and the like than to accept any philosophical theory which claims we cannot know or reasonably believe or reasonably securely accept that we may not do such things.[14] Some, perhaps all, of these moral truisms, as I like to call them, are things which are only **ceteris paribus** wrong. This means that in some at least imaginable circumstances they can, as a lesser evil, be done but that notwithstanding there **always** is a **presumption** against doing them. (In the case of torturing the innocent that standing presumption is very stringent indeed.) What is crucial to keep before our minds here is that there is always a standing presumption against doing these things. We know, or can reasonably believe or accept, that these things are at least in this way wrong and that it is more reasonable to accept this claim than to accept a skeptical ethical theory that tells us that we can never know or are never justified in believing or accepting that anything is right or wrong.[15]

However, this "critical commonsensist" breaking of ethical skepticism—or at least a certain conception of ethical skepticism—is of no help to the applied ethicist claiming ethical expertise. The knowledge of right and wrong we have here—if "knowledge" is the right word for it—is something that is perfectly available to every statistically normal human being; this knowledge of right or wrong (the first-order claim of it) is not something that we could reasonably claim to have as a matter of **expertise**. It is not derived from a meta-ethical theory or grounded in a normative ethical theory or any combination of them and in fact it is used by many philosophers as one crucial test of the adequacy of normative ethical theories. That is to say, it has a fundamental place in theory-acceptance.[16]

However, such a Moorean turn, while it is cogent against an ethical skepticism (if such there be) that tells us we can never reasonably believe or accept that anything is right or wrong or a skepticism that tells us that moral beliefs are all illusions, is not effective against the moral skepticism I discussed above. (That in fact was the kind of ethical skepticism that had such a thorough articulation and defense in the work of Westermarck.[17]) Traditional normative moralists, as Edward Westermarck called them, set out to develop theories which would rationalize our moral beliefs and give us a systematic knowledge of right and wrong with a supreme principle or consistent set of principles of morality and a way of deriving, in some senses of that term, lower level principles or rules—maxims of the mid-level—that would (together with more general principles and a knowledge of the facts) systematically guide and rationalize our practices and actions. But it is not at all clear that we have any such systematic moral knowledge or that moral philosophers can reasonably expect that their Newton will someday come along. It is not even clear that we have a defensible or even a coherent account of a "true morality" or a "true moral perspective." My Moorean turn against a certain kind of skepticism has done nothing to allay my previous skepticism about whether we have--or are on the verge of acquiring--some systematic knowledge of right and wrong such that this could supply the theoretical under-pinning for applied ethics, giving the ethicist the wherewithal to acquire the ethical expertise that could legitimate their activity and establish their authority. I have tried to give reasons for being skeptical that applied ethicists have available anything like this.

V

Even with a reasonable conception of moral progress intact the above situation would not be altered. Ruth Macklin has use-usefully displayed criteria for moral progress such that some-times we can make some rough ranking of societies, at least when their economic conditions of life are roughly similar.[18] Working with the ordinary meanings of our evaluative terms "humane" and "human" (evaluative in some contexts), Macklin articulates what she calls "the principle of humaneness" and "the principle of humanity." These two principles, she argues, yield criteria of moral progress. The **principle of humaneness** tells us that one "culture, society or historical era exhibits a higher degree of moral progress than another if the first shows more sensitivity to (less tolerance of) the pain and suffering of human beings than does the second, as expressed in the laws, customs, institutions, and practices of the respective societies or eras."[19] The **principle of humanity** reads: "One culture, society or historical era exhibits a higher degree of moral progress than another if the first shows more recognition of the inherent dignity, the basic autonomy, or the intrinsic worth of human beings than does the second as expressed in the laws, customs, institutions, and practices of the respective societies or eras."[20] The key conceptions here, as Macklin is well aware, are vague and some of them are perhaps essentially contested. **Sometimes** they would be difficult to apply. In comparing society or practice x with society or practice y, it would not infrequently be difficult to say which satisfied these criteria more adequately. Sometimes in comparing practices or institutions, let alone whole societies, it is difficult to ascertain the degree of pain and suffering but often it is perfectly evident, e.g. Sweden in 1944 compared with Germany in 1944, Yugoslavia in 1982 compared with Chile in 1982 or Cuba in 1982 compared with Haiti in 1982. We also need to keep in mind that concepts such as "inherent dignity" or "intrinsic worth" will be given at least partially different readings in different normative ethical theories and their criteria are not (to put it minimally) completely agreed upon. Some very iconoclastic theories will even challenge their coherence. Though note we

103

would have to go rather far afield for such examples. Even Nietzsche was not unambivalent about such conceptions. Moreover, they are not for us like the concept of taboo is alleged to have been for the Polynesians when they were visited by Captain Cook. Still, we do not agree about the elucidation of the concepts of intrinsic worth, autonomy and dignity and some of us may even see them (or at least some of them) as being in some degree metaphorical or hyperbolic, but our criteria of application are not so indefinite as not to make it perfectly evident that the inherent dignity or intrinsic worth of persons was not honored in Belsen, is not being honored when right-wing death squads round up peasants and intellectuals in Latin America and is not being honored for many of the residents of Harlem or South Chicago. That we cannot make fine discriminations about practices, institutions or societies does not mean that cruder but still humanly speaking vital discriminations cannot be firmly made.

We indeed must make these judgments with a sense of historical and cultural context, though this does not imply an acceptance of any of the wellknown forms of relativism. To achieve moral balance and to avoid a superficial utopianism here, we also need something like Fredrick Engels' grim and chastening recognition that "Without slavery, no Greek state, no Greek art and science; without slavery no Roman Empire. But without Hellenism and the Roman Empire...no modern Europe." To be serious about morality, we need unblindly to recognize, as both Engels and Marx did, the unavoidability of hard conditions and the necessity of long and bitter historically conditioned struggles for human emancipation. We need to hold this unsettling or at least saddening fact in balance and square it with, as both Engels and Marx did, our intuitive (pre-theoretical) moral belief that moral progress is crucially "exhibited in the gradual abolition of slavery and the prohibition of cruel and unusual punishment in the history of penal and judicial practices."[21] But we do not need a fancy moral theory or indeed any theory at all, to recognize that or to tell us that in life the moral choice is not infrequently some agonizing choice of a lesser evil.[22]

A significant thing about Macklin's principles is that they yield criteria of moral progress and are themselves principles that are not dependent on the acceptance of any of the rival competing objectivist normative ethical theories. One could be utterly agnostic about or even dismissive of the very possibility of a normative ethical theory and still accept the principle of humaneness and the principle of humanity. Even Edward Westermarck, in the face of the thoroughness and extent of his rejection of ethical objectivism, quite self-consciously operated with such principles in viewing different societies.[23] Remember he was a social evolutionist utilizing the comparative method in social anthropology as well as a defender of what he called eth-

ical relativism.[24] Only a skeptic or nihilist whose skepticism
or nihilism ran so deep, or became so paradoxical, as to run
afoul of my Moorean strictures, would not, at least in effect,
accept something rather like Macklin's principles of humaneness
and humanity with their entailed criteria of moral progress. But
acceptance of such principles does not commit one to the acceptance of any moral theory at all or even to the belief in the
very possibility of a normative ethical theory. Westermarck
quite consistently rejected normative moralism while accepting
the principles of humaneness and humanity. (I do not say that
Westermarck explicitly articulated such principles but that an
examination of his work shows that he in effect assumed such
conceptions.[25])

The acceptance of these principles does not ground any claim
to moral expertise or yield a justified belief in the viability
of "applied ethics" with its mid-level moral rules. A person who
would accept considered judgments such as the ones mentioned in
my Moorean strategy could readily be persuaded to accept at least
something like the principle of humaneness and the principle of
humanity. And, if we do not start from such firm considered judgments and indeed return to them at crucial moments in a quest for
justification, it is· very difficult to know where we could start
or where we could touch base in asking what it is we are to
believe morally.[26] But the having of that starting point and the
utilization of that vindication-criterion requires no moral expertise or other philosophical expertise and the beliefs and understanding requisite for the reflective acceptance of the principles of humaneness and humanity, and hence of some minimal
conception of moral progress and objectivity, do not require it
either.

VI

It is not unnatural to say that I have neglected one of the
key things that a philosophically informed ethics can, and sometimes does, achieve. It can contribute greater clarity to what
would otherwise be a more intuitive, helter-skelter facing of
concrete social problems. Philosophers, and other philosophically literate intellectuals, can, by using their analytical
skills, clarify, sometimes in important ways, crucial social
issues and can, in this way, provide the expertise we require for
the developing of an applied ethics. At the very least, they can
function as conceptual or logical policemen sniffing out invalid
arguments and the like.

It is hard to knock clarity and plainly it is something we
should prize and seek to cultivate. Yet we should not make a
fetish out of it and, particularly if we are philosophers, who
also somehow think of ourselves as ethicists, we should be very
cautious in our claims concerning the wonders it can work. It is

important, of course, to spot invalid arguments, particularly when their invalidity could be corrected by a little inessential tinkering. But sometimes a concern for clarity comes to little more than pedantry or to the taking of baroque means to rationalize what we prefer to believe or perhaps even very much need to believe. Alternatively, it can come to finding neat distinctions and conceptualizations to defend one side or another in some social debate where the essential terms of the debate are never questioned by either side.

Considerable ingenuity is often expended in such philosophical discussions on remaining normatively neutral. If we can only draw, it is often implicitly assumed, clear distinctions between kinds of paternalism, indoctrination, community, conceptions of what intrinsic goodness or ethical rationality come to and the like, we will at last be able to resolve or dissolve many of our central moral perplexities, without ever taking a moral or political stance at all or at least without trotting out anything other than the barest commonplaces concerning which there is a very considerable consensus.

Sometimes clarification does help, sometimes people in the midst of moral dispute are simply confused and when the confusion is brought home to them they will abandon even a fairly deeply entrenched particular moral belief. But, perhaps more typically, the clarification will only enable the disputants to define their differences a little more clearly; or, worse, it will only equip them with a new or somewhat more streamlined jargon in which to display their differences; or worse still, it will track them off into a barren debate about rather abstract issues far from the specific social moral issue with which they were trying to come to grips in the first instance. Sometimes what the normative issue is in some social conflict is not clear; sometimes, in an amorphous but at least seemingly important social conflict, a normative issue needs to get forged in demanding and disciplined intellectual discussion. But often the clarification will not help the contestants gain new moral knowledge or even provide them with an aid toward gaining a more perspicuous representation of "the foundations" of that knowledge. If the ethicist does not have a profound understanding of human history, culture and psychology, it is rather unlikely that his clarifications will come to much, will be of much value in gaining a better understanding of the moral life or help us very much in the difficult task of moral and cultural criticism. I think Cheryl Noble's twitting of a certain non-atypical moral philosopher's assumption of ethical expertise is very much to the point: "the would-be critic," she remarks, "who does not understand the economic and psychological pushes and pulls on moral thinking lacks the kind of self-consciousness which is the precondition for being able to think critically."[27]

VII

There is a more general point that needs to be understood and taken to heart. Once a philosophically oriented commitment to analysis and clarification was clearly linked to an overall philosophical programme with an emancipatory intent. Today such a programme is far more problematical. Richard Rorty has noted an important difference here between positivist and post-positivist analytical philosophy. For Hans Reichenbach (and similar things could be said of Russell, Ayer, or Popper and even in a way of Austin) the commitment to clarity through analysis was linked with a meta-philosophy which aimed at giving us something like a scientific philosophy which would replace grandiose philosophical speculation and system building with a philosophical activity which, as the analytic handmaiden of science, would provide us with a rigorously argued scientific world-perspective.[28] But, as post-positivist analytic philosophy, in at least a seemingly cummulative series of shifts, slowly thrusts itself on our consciousness—I am thinking here principally of the rather diverse work of Wittgenstein, Austin, Quine and Sellars—the "powerful analytic tools" that Reichenbach so prized turned out to be indefensible positivistic dogmas or at least highly tendentious philosophical theses concerning which there is no philosophical, let alone, scientific consensus.[29]

As this development of analytic philosophy accelerated and the wheel churning out new philosophical theories sped up and the new theories proliferated into an embarrassment of local dialects, it became increasingly evident that the analytic successors to the positivists had neither left us with a meta-philosophy nor with a distinctive philosophical programme. There is nothing, in post-positivist analytical philosophy, identifiable as a philosophical method, which would give us a perspicuous representation of our concepts or of our various forms of life. Likewise there is nothing identifiable as "applied philosophy" (say biomedical ethics) affording us a clear and critical analysis of our practical problems or giving us a framework which would move us in the direction of their resolution, through an enhanced understanding and a perspicuous display and critical probing of our concepts. Post-positivist analytical philosophy in short gave us no distinctive philosophical basis for a critical ethics. Instead the expertise of the post-positivist analytical philosopher is, as Richard Rorty has nicely put it, more like that of a lawyer.[30] Such a philosopher works with cases, develops the capacity to construct a good brief, conduct a devastating cross-examination, see clearly a large number of inferential relationships and provide, like a good sophist, an argument for any kind of substantive position. While for Hans Reichenbach or Bertrand Russell or Ernest Nagel, there was a commitment to clarity in the service of a scientific world-perspective, for post-positivist analytic philosophers, there is no clear rationale for their clarification: there is no philosophical knowledge to be gained, no demarcation of science from metaphysics or ideology to be drawn, no systematic representation of our concepts to be constructed or critique of our society to be made. Post-positivist analytical philosophers afford us no hope of the gaining of a framework from which such a critique could be carried out. There is no clear conception of what the demand for clarity should come to. I grant that, even without such an understanding, occasionally, in some specific situations, a demand for clarity can have a not inconsiderable value. But it can also stand in the way of our moral appreciation of what is at issue in actual moral conflicts and it can deflect a perfectly reasonable and necessary resolve to act. Moreover, it is not clear in general what a demand for clarity comes to. We have no coherent conception of what "complete clarity," particularly in such nonformal domains, would consist in. In such a milieu, talk of "applied ethics" becomes something which is very anomalous indeed.

One does not need to be committed to an engineering model for "applied ethics" (something aptly criticized by Arthur Caplan) to recognize that if physics totters applied physics does as well and that if philosophy becomes problematic moral philosophy, then applied ethics does so as well.[31] But analytic philosophy, in the ways I have just described, has become either problematic or pedestrian with little emancipatory potential and it is far from clear whether we have any plausible conception or even reasonable hunch of what its successors would look like.[32] But "an applied ethics," as its very name indicates, is not an independent activity. And it looks like it has no philosophical basis or at least none is clearly in sight. Perhaps, we could and should have "applied ethics without philosophy." But then what is its rationale? Are we seriously going to suggest going to theology? But even a passing acquaintance with the state of the art there is hardly something to encourage a sober-minded and reflective person.[33] However, if not theology then what? Should we try out some smelly ideology?

I think we should try out the utilization of a certain range of a certain kind of critical social science or social theory. But this is the topic for a less nay-saying occasion.[34] It must have, to be anything other than programmatic hot air, a reasonably clear articulation and elaboration and the proof of this new pudding is indeed in the eating. That is to say, we must be able to show how it can systematically resolve a fair number of practical moral issues. Moreover, we must also be able to show that it has theoretical resources beyond that of plain reflective common sense. It is, in fact, what has become fashionable to call, a new research program and it should be viewed with a not inconsiderable suspicion. But my effort here was not the programmatic statement of that constructive task but to argue that

traditional approaches to applied ethics, including biomedical
ethics, are in shambles.

FOOTNOTES

[1] I am not fond of such terminology. But such talk has got into the literature.

[2] Edward Westermarck, THE ORIGIN AND DEVELOPMENT OF THE MORAL IDEAS, 2 volumes (London: Macmillan Co., 1906-8), and ETHICAL RELATIVITY (London: Kegan Paul, 1932). See the discussions of Westermarck, including my own, in EDWARD WESTERMARCK: ESSAYS ON HIS LIFE AND WORKS (ACTA PHILOSOPHICA FENNICA) Vol. 33, (1982) ed. Timothy Stroup. See also Apex Hagerstrom, PHILOSOPHY AND RELIGION, trans. Robert Sandin (London: Allen and Unwin, 1964), pp. 77-172 and John Anderson, STUDIES IN EMPIRICAL PHILOSOPHY (Sydney, Australia: Angus and Robertson, 1962), pp. 214-374. J. L. Mackie, H. D. Munro and Gilbert Harman are important but still derivative figures here: J. L. Mackie, ETHICS: INVENTING RIGHT AND WRONG (Harmondsworth, Middlesex, England: Penguin Books, 1977); D. H. Monro, EMPIRICISM AND ETHICS (Cambridge, England: Cambridge University Press, 1967) and Gilbert Harman, THE NATURE OF MORALITY (New York: Oxford University Press, 1977).

[3] Alan Gewrith, REASON AND MORALITY (Chicago: University of Chicago Press, 1978). I have developed more extensively my critique of Gewirth in "Against Ethical Rationalism" in GEWIRTH'S ETHICAL RATIONALISM, ed. Edward Regis, Jr. (Chicago: University of Chicago Press, 1983). There are two, perhaps natural, but still mistaken, readings of my arguments in this section and indeed of the entire thrust of my essay that I would like to block. (1) I am not in search, let alone in a des-despairing search, of an ultimate moral theory: the one "true morality" that would apply for all time and in all places. In criticizing Rawl's claimed Archimedian point, I share his overall fallibility. (We can grow into a fallibility without any residue of a nostalgia for the Absolute.) I seek no stronger Archimedian point than a standpoint (a perspective) which would give us (people living in a technologically advanced world under conditions of moderate scarcity or what could be conditions of moderate scarcity) a set of principles such that properly informed rational agents in such a world, unfettered by the constructions of a particular culture and a particular ideological indoctrination, would come by way of a consensus to accept these principles and would come to accept, as well, a procedure (a methodology, if you will) which, along with the principles, would be of sufficient cogency to enable us validly to assess social practices and ways of responding to one another. The principles and procedures would be accepted by way of a consensus obtaining among such rational agents under conditions that Habermas describes as those of unconstrained communication. I would also require that the principles and procedures be of sufficient strength to give us a similarly accepted account of

progress in moral understanding and in moral theory (including an acceptance that there is such progress and a consensus concerning its general direction). We have (**pace** Feyerabend) something like this in science. We have, that is, some conception of a progressive development in science. But it does not seem to me evident that we have it either in ethics or in ethical theory. (2) In criticizing Rawls, I do not reject, as some have thought, his method of wide reflective equilibrium. I think, though not without ambivalence, that the application of that method in a certain way is the best hope we have in ethical theory in trying to develop a method for theory acceptance and theory assessment and in seeking criteria for assessing moral practices and moralities. What I have criticized, in various places, is Rawls' own articulation of a set of principles of justice displayed in lexical order. I have argued that these principles do not give us an acceptable Archimedian point and I have also criticized Rawls' contractarian method and what I take to be his background ideological assumptions. But, I would like to note here that, even if we accept his method of wide reflective equilibrium, this will not **ipso facto** commit us to a belief in a rational development in morality or of moral theory or show that such a consensus in fact obtains. But I do not think this is an **a priori** matter or that it is something over which it is reasonably evident that Rawls is mistaken. In fine, I am aware that it remains very much a matter of controversy with a considerable amount of sorting out yet to be done. See notes 5, 16, 22 and 26 for the citations appropriate to this note.

[4] In what sense Rawls is and in what sense he is not a Kantian is clearly enough expressed in his John Dewey lectures. see "Kantian Constructivism in Moral Theory," THE JOURNAL OF PHILOSOPHY 77(September, 1980), pp. 515-572 and A THEORY OF JUSTICE (Cambridge, Mass.: Harvard University Press, 1971), pp. 251-257 and 445.

[5] The critiques of Rawls are legion and they reflect a variety of philosophical and ideological perspectives. The following five volumes collect together usefully a range of criticisms of Rawls: Norman Daniels, ed., READING RAWLS, (New York: Basic Books, 1975); Kai Nielsen and Roger Shiner, eds., NEW ESSAYS ON CONTRACT THEORY (Guelph, Ontario: Canadian Association for Publishing in Philosophy, 1977); John Arthur and William Shaw, eds., JUSTICE AND ECONOMIC DISTRIBUTION (Englewood Cliffs, NJ: Prentice-Hall, 1978); H. Gene Blocker and Elizabeth Smith, eds., JOHN RAWLS' THEORY OF SOCIAL JUSTICE (Athens, Ohio: Ohio University Press, 1980); and the issue of THE OCCASIONAL REVIEW, Issue 8/9 (Autumn 1978) devoted to an examination of Rawls and Nozick. For two important recent critiques and overviews of Rawls see Gerald Doppelt, "Rawls' System of Justice: A Critique from the Left," NOUS 15 (September, 1981), pp. 295-307, and Brian Barry, "Critical Notice of Wolff: Under-

standing Rawls" CANADIAN JOURNAL OF PHILOSOPHY 8(Dec., 1978), pp. 753-784. There is a useful bibliography of writings on Rawls at the end of my "Morality and Ideology: Some Radical Critiques of Rawls," GRADUATE FACULTY PHILOSOPHY JOURNAL 8(Spring, 1982), pp. 189-267. I think a careful study of these various critiques will reveal two things (1) the complexity, reflective sophistication and systematic power of Rawls' book, together with its astute awareness of difficulties and alternatives in the history of moral thought and (2) that notwithstanding, it will reveal the critical undermining of the central pillars of his account. For my own various critiques of Rawls see the above cited bibliography pp. 260-262.

[6]Alasdair MacIntyre sets out his critique of contemporary moral philosophy in "A Crisis in Moral Philosophy: Why is the Search for the Foundations of Ethics so Frustrating?" in THE ROOTS OF ETHICS, ed. Daniel Callahan and H. Tristram Engelhardt, Jr. (New York: Plenum Press, 1981), pp. 3-20. This polemical programmatic includes a brusque dismissal of Rawls. Gerald Dworkin, in the same volume, effectively argues that this critique of Rawls is misdirected. But that does not prevent MacIntyre's overall picture of the ills of moral theory from being challenging. However, his major work here (and the one I criticize above) is AFTER VIRTUE (Notre Dame, Indiana: Notre Dame University Press, 1981).

[7]MacIntyre's book has received a lot of praise in general journals and cultural reviews. For a typical such essay, but still one which also has the merit of clearly, accurately and in some detail setting out MacIntyre's views, see Cameron "Can We Live the Good Life?," NEW YORK REVIEW OF BOOKS 28(November 5, 1981), pp. 44-48. For a severely critical examination which is, I believe, also very much to the point, see Simon Blackburn, "Critical Notice: AFTER VIRTUE," PHILOSOPHICAL INVESTIGATIONS, 5(April, 1982), pp. 146-154. Unlike many of the discussions in the cultural reviews, Blackburn comes neither to praise nor to situate MacIntyre but carefully to assess his account.

[8]Andrew Levine and Erik Wright, "Rationality and Class Struggle," NEW LEFT REVIEW, 123(Sept.-Oct.,1980), pp. 47-68; Agnes Heller, THE THEORY OF NEED IN MARX (London: Allison and Busby, 1974), and "Can 'true' and 'false' Needs be Posited?" in HUMAN NEEDS: A CONTRIBUTION TO THE CURRENT DEBATE, ed. Katrim Lederer (Cambridge, Mass.: Oelgeschlager, Gunn and Hain, 1980), pp. 213-226; and Patricia Springborg, THE PROBLEM OF HUMAN NEEDS AND THE CRITIQUE OF CIVILISATION (London: Allen and Unwin, 1981).

[9] Alasdair MacIntyre develops his conception of essentially contextual concepts in "The Essential Contestability of Some Social Concepts," ETHICS 84(Oct., 1973), pp. 1-9.

[10] I continue to use the sexist vocabulary of the English translations of Aristotle.

[11] See Rawls' account of the primary social goods in A THEORY OF JUSTICE, pp. 90-95.

[12] See the reference in Note 1.

[13] H. D. Munro, "Relativism in Ethics," DICTIONARY OF THE HISTORY OF IDEAS, vol. IV, ed. Philip Wiener (New York: Scribner, 1973), pp. 70-74.

[14] It is essential to leave those alternatives intact to stay on tolerably secure grounds.

[15] It is salutory to ask if any of the skeptical moral theories, theories which give to understand that the search for (the true morality) or even a true morality is a Holmesless Watson, would really claim anything that strong. I doubt if any of these skeptical moral philosophers would bite that bullet any more than David Hume would. If my doubt is well directed, the next question is, what, if any, moral should we draw from that? It looks a bit as if something has gone wrong here.

[16] Rawls, A THEORY OF JUSTICE, pp. 46-53, 201, 577-587 and "Independence of Moral Theory," PROCEEDINGS AND ADDRESSES OF THE AMERICAN PHILOSOPHICAL ASSOCIATION 48(1974-5) pp. 5-22. Also see the following four important articles by Norman Daniels: "Wide Reflective Equilibrium and Theory Acceptance in Ethics," THE JOURNAL OF PHILOSOPHY 76(May, 1979), pp. 256-282; "Moral Theory and the Plasticity of Persons," THE MONIST 62(July, 1979), pp. 265-287; "Reflective Equilibrium and Archimedian Points," CANADIAN JOURNAL OF PHILOSOPHY, 10(March, 1980), pp. 83-103; and "On Some Methods of Ethics and Linguistics," PHILOSOPHICAL STUDIES 37(January, 1980), pp. 21-36.

[17] See the reference to Westermarck in note 2. The classic criticism--I did not say a justified criticism--is given by G. E. Moore in PHILOSOPHICAL STUDIES (New York: Humanities Press, 1951), pp. 331-339. For an accurate and sympathetic account of Westermarck which shows how his account is not touched by these traditional criticisms see Timothy Stroup, "In Defense of Westermarck," JOURNAL OF THE HISTORY OF PHILOSOPHY 19(April, 1981), pp. 213-234.

[18] Ruth Macklin, "Moral Progress," ETHICS 87(1977), pp. 370-372.

[19] Ibid., pp. 372 and 375.

[20] Ibid.

[21] Ibid., p. 372.

[22] Michael Teitelman, "On the Theory of the Practice of the Theory of Justice," JOURNAL OF CHINESE PHILOSOPHY 5(1978), pp. 217-247.

[23] Westermarck, THE ORIGIN AND DEVELOPMENT OF THE MORAL IDEAS (Volume I), pp. 12, 60-1, 119-20, 122-24, 131, 158, 182, 201-2, 214-37,273-75,283-4, 300, 312-13, (Vol. II), 176-74, 226-28, 738, 741-46. There are similar passages in his ETHICAL RELATIVITY, pp. 46, 76-7, 112,, 146-7, 160-61,163, 200, 217, 253. These various passages show that Westermarck, in spite of his avowed ethical subjectivism, has an important though submerged conception of objectivity that did not depend on accepting ethical realism and involved centrally a firm conception of a gradually developing enlightenment moral consciousness.

[24] Edward Westermarck, "Methods in Social Anthropology," THE JOURNAL OF THE ROYAL ANTHROPOLOGICAL INSTITUTE OF GREAT BRITAIN AND IRELAND 66(1936), pp. 223-248. A deep ambivalence about social evolution and about some uses of some form of the comparative method in contemporary social anthropology is much in evidence in E. E. Evans-Pritchard's, A HISTORY OF ANTHROPOLOGICAL THOUGHT (London: Farbar and Farber, 1981).

[25] See the references in footnote 23. The page references there are crucial.

[26] See my papers, "On Needing a Moral Theory," METAPHILOSOPHY 13(April, 1983), pp. 97-116; "Grounding Rights and a Method of Reflective Equilibrium," INQUIRY, forthcoming; "Reason and Sentiment" in RATIONALITY TODAY, ed. T. Gaerets (Ottawa, Canada: University of Ottawa Press, 1979), pp. 249-279; "Considered Judgments," RATIO 19(June, 1977), pp. 39-46; and "Considered Judgments Again," HUMAN STUDIES 5(April-June, 1982), pp. 109-118.

[27] Cheryl Noble, "Response," THE HASTINGS CENTER REPORT, 12(June, 1982), p. 15. The exchange between Noble and her critics "Ethics and Experts" in the above issue of the journal is an instructive one as far as the issues discussed in this essay are concerned. Noble's case about applied ethics and ethical theory is in certain respects like mine. But she overstates her case in certain respects and thus makes herself unnecessarily vulnerable to her critics. In particular, Daniel Wikler, in his judicious response, makes points that a balanced account would

have to incorporate. Singer and Beauchamp, on the other hand, ethics and ethical experts.

[28]Richard Rorty, "Philosophy in America," THE AMERICAN SCHOLAR (1982).

[29]Hans Reichenbach, THE RISE OF SCIENTIFIC PHILOSOPHY 11(December, 1981), pp. 569-589.

[30]Rorty, "Philosophy in America."

[31]Arthur Caplan, "Applying Morality to Advances in Biomedicine: Can and Should this be Done" in NEW KNOWLEDGE IN THE BIOMEDICAL SCIENCES, ed. William Bondeson et al. (Dordrecht, Holland: Reidel, 1982), pp. 155-168.

[32]I am not here suggesting that things are better ordered on the Continent. The difficulties are different but they are at least as considerable.

[33]Perhaps this sounds dogmatic? But see my IN DEFENSE OF ATHEISM, (Buffalo, New York: Prometheus Books, 1983) and "God and the Basis of Morality," JOURNAL OF RELIGIOUS ETHICS, 10(Fall, 1982), pp. 335-350.

[34]Some of the programme is suggested in my "Critical Theory, Social Science and Values," LIBERAL AND FINE ARTS REVIEW, forthcoming 1983, and in my "Emancipatory Social Science and Social Critique" in ETHICS, THE SOCIAL SCIENCES AND POLICY ANALYSIS, ed. Daniel Callahan and Bruce Jennings (New York, Plenum Press, 1983).

ON BEING A CASUIST

Albert R. Jonsen

Ethical theory has come under heavy criticism in this conference. Arthur Caplan and Kai Nielsen have both expressed
skepticism about its adequacy, both in itself and as a useful
guide in practical ethics.[1,2] One of the co-directors of this
conference also has repudiated ethical theory as a source of bioethical evaluation. He describes the view which he repudiates as
"the attempt to articulate the logical implications of a principle arrived at in general moral theory for some set of biomedical
situations."[3] Yet, working with ethical theory--devising it,
refining it, criticizing it, reconstructing it and drawing conclusions from it--is the moral philosopher's metier; many moral
philosophers are committed to the rigor and elegance of system
and theory. Jonathan Glover, for example, writes of the "aesthe-
tic preference most of us have for economy of principle, a
preference for ethical systems in the style of Bauhaus rather
than the Baroque."[4]

If ethical theory is inadequate or inappropriate for the
task of practical ethics, how is practical ethics to be done? Is
there an alternative to "ethics demonstrated in geometric
fashion"?[5] I propose that there is and that it is in the Baroque
rather than the Bauhaus style. Indeed, it is not merely Baroque
in the metaphorical sense of being elaborate rather than elegant,
riotous rather than rigorous; it is Baroque in the historical
sense of having been created and having flourished during the
Baroque era of European Civilization. The alternative way to do
practical ethics is casuistry.[6]

Casuistry has been, to say the least, out of fashion for
several centuries. The Oxford English Dictionary defines the
word as "a quibbling or evasive way of dealing with difficult
questions of duty," gives "sophistry" as a synonym and quotes an
18th century author, "casuistry destroys, by distinctions and
exceptions, all morality and effaces the difference between right
and wrong." The great moral philosopher Sidgwick put it more
delicately: ". . . casuistry has a tendency to weaken the moral
sensibilities of ordinary minds."[6,7] Strange, is it not, that
with such a reputation, casuistry seems to be coming back into
fashion. It is a truism in bioethics that one should focus on
cases and that teaching is best done through cases. Certain
cases, like Quinlan, Saikewicz, and Baby Doe of Bloomington, are
rehearsed in learned exchanges between the applied ethicists.
Texts and readers are crammed with cases. More and more, one
hears the tentative, somewhat embarrassed suggestion that a "new
casuistry is needed." Indeed, the staunchest champion of principle, Paul Ramsey, has written approvingly:

Medical ethics today must, indeed, be a
casuistry; it must deal as competently and
exhaustively as possible with the concrete
features of actual moral decisions of life
and death and medical care.[8]

Could it be that the practice so scathingly condemned by the
genius Pascal in 1665 as "scandalous and excessive moral license,
shameful and pernicious moral teaching"[9] is about to become
respectable again? I think it is and I will tell you how, in my
opinion, a casuistry should be done.

I am a casuist and not at all ashamed of it. In my work as
an educator of medical students and graduate physicians, I do
casuistry daily. With Mark Siegler and William Winslade, I
produced CLINICAL ETHICS, which is a casuistical handbook.[10]
As a Commissioner on the National Commission for the Protection
of Human Subjects of Biomedical and Behavioral Research, I spent
four years working out the ethics of research with human subjects.
Stephen Toulmin, who was consultant to the Commission, and I
realized, to our astonishment, that the Commission was engaged in
a sustained casuistry.[11] As a result of that experience, we are
preparing a history, methodology, and, in a certain sense, a
theory of casuistry. Finally, I was trained as a Jesuit. Though
Jesuitry and casuistry share the same opprobrious connotations,
with some good reason, it is historically true that, during the
16th and 17th centuries, the Jesuits were skilled practitioners
of casuistry in the sense which Toulmin and I believe is a positive, fruitful way of thinking about moral issues. I am, then,
going to be a casuist in this paper. I will present a case, do
some casuistry with it, and reflect on the elements which Toulmin
and I consider the essence of the casuistic method and which dif-
ferentiates this method from the methods of modern moral philosophy and applied ethics.

The Case

Being a casuist is a bit like being a cynic, a stoic, or a
pragmatist. One can either be thought of as having certain
characteristics of attitude and behavior which merit the epithet
or one can be quite explicitly identified with those persons who
associated themselves historically with the development and propa-
gation of a certain doctrine. There were Cynics, Stoics, and
Pragmatists; living, breathing teachers and pupils in actual
"schools of thought." So were there Casuists: persons who did
casuistry as their daily occupation, as it were. Mostly, though
not exclusively, Roman Catholic theologians, philosophers and
jurists, they flourished from about 1450 to 1850. They produced
many books, filled with myriad cases of moral perplexity ranging
from issues of high public policy to personal problems. They
collected in their tomes what we today separate into distinct

118

fields of sociology, political science, economics, psychology, philosophy and theology. They engaged in intense communication through the printed book, citing and criticizing each other's opinions in successive editions. On some subjects such as usury, major debates raged over long years, finally reaching agreement with precise areas of disagreement. Casuistry was, in its time, a bit like "Washington Week in Review" or "Agronsky and Company," carried on through the cooler medium of the book.

At about the midpoint of its heyday, the brilliant mathematician, physicist, and religious mystic, Blaise Pascal, produced a scathing critique of casuistry, **THE PROVINCIAL LETTERS**, which stands still as a masterpiece of French literature. This critique, done for complex reasons which we will not rehearse, was to some extent justified, but its sarcasm withered not only the excesses of casuistry but the entire endeavor, giving it as a whole the bad name it carries today.

Pascal was particularly revolted by a case which he quotes from his favorite casuist, the Jesuit Escobar. I will use this case as my own example for the rest of this paper, calling it, "The Case of the Contemned Captain." Here is Escobar:

> A noble may kill someone who has slapped him
> even if that person runs away, provided that
> he avoid doing so out of hatred or vengeance,
> thus giving no occasion for these excessive
> murders so harmful to society. The reason is
> that one may run after one's honour, as one
> does after stolen goods. For, although your
> honour is not in the hands of your enemy,
> like property he might have stolen, yet it
> may be recovered in the same way, by showing
> signs of dignity and authority and thus
> acquiring public esteem. It is not true that
> anyone who has been slapped is reputed dis-
> honored until he has killed his enemy.[12]

Pascal found this "a horrible and damnable doctrine," as I am sure the reader agrees. This antique example will, however, illustrate our propositions about the nature of casuistry. I will offer five such propositions, under the headings "Paradigm and Analogy," "Circumstances," "Maxims," "Arguability," and "Resolution." Each of these represents a peculiar feature of classical casuistry and, in a significant way, distinguishes casuistry from contemporary moral philosophy.

Paradigm and Analogy

Outrageous though it is, we must view the Case of the Contemned Captain in its context. It had appeared in books of casuistry some fifty years before Escobar cited it, and it was argued for another half-century until condemned by papal decree as one of several hundred casuistic opinions which ecclesiastical authorities deemed "scandalous." The case is situated within an exposition of the fifth commandment of the Decalogue, "Thou shalt not kill." The casuists move from paradigms, cases in which a moral maxim was clearly applicable, to analogies, cases in which, due to different circumstances, a maxim appeared less suitable, more open to rebuttal, more susceptible to exception. In this treatise, the paradigm case would be instances in which the moral maxim of the Commandment is most clearly and unambiguously appropriate: the intentional killing of an innocent person. The case of killing in warfare would follow, then the case of defense of one's life against attack, defense of others' lives, of one's property, one's virtue, and, finally, of one's honor. As cases were constructed, the casuists recognized that the justification of killing in defense of one's life when under attack moves from a highly plausible to a much less plausible argument when other goods than life are at stake. At the time Escobar states this case, the defense of honor was considered at least arguable. The movement from paradigm to analogy, that is, from more obvious application of moral maxim to less obvious ones, is one of the principal characteristics of classical casuistry.

Circumstances

A theologian much revered by the casuists, Thomas Aquinas, wrote, "human actions should be considered differently in view of different conditions of person, time and other circumstances."[13] The casuists, instructed by a decree of the Church which required confessors "to inquire diligently into the circumstances of the sin and of the sinner," set out a list of circumstances, adopted from the classical rhetoricians, "who, what, where, by what means, why, how and when" (Lateran IV, 1215).[14] They treated circumstances most seriously, for it is not that circumstances merely alter cases, as the old saying goes: circumstances **make** cases. It is the set of concrete facts extant in an instance that allows it to be said, "this is a case of killing, this is a case of self defense," etc., and to rehearse the arguments appropriate to cases of that sort.

The case of the contemned captain was one of those cases which, as I mentioned, was debated by many casuists over many years. During the course of the debate, authors expatiated on the circumstances: the person of honor is "a captain of the king's guard," "a person of great public eminence,"; the insult takes place in private or in the presence of other nobles, legal means of redress are at hand or are not; the insult is almost an assault, etc. In this juggling of circumstances, they are after an important question: how far away is the defense of honor from

120

what is, in this area of morality, a primary paradigm, namely, defense of one's life against a direct physical attack.

Can honor be considered as good as one's life? Some casuists note that, for those whose lives are deeply affected by reputation and esteem of the people, it might be. For monks, whose life is humility, it certainly is not so. One casuist remarks, "slaps and thrashing are certainly not offensive to common folk." Is honor like property, as Escobar asserts? Some casuists remark the officer of the king's guard makes a living out of a reputation for fierce bravery: honor is, in a sense, his livelihood. Behind these comments, which seem so strange to us, is a cultural conception of reputation and honor which we do not share (except where Sicilian "respetta" still prevails). It is fascinating to see, over the one hundred years of the debate, a fading of the chivalric honor which still flourished in the late 16th century Spain; indeed, one casuist, an Austrian, notes that this opinion could plausibly be held only in Spain.

The plausibility of interpreting honor as equivalent to personal identity or to property is profoundly conditioned by the culture: honor is a convention. As the casuists perceive this, they also preceive that the analogy with the primary paradigm of self defense is a very weak one. Thus, circumstances determine not only the moral species, as the casuist said, but also the strength or weakness of the analogy in relation to the more primary paradigms. At the end of the debate, casuists were saying, "this is not a case of self defense. It is nothing more than a case of foolish vainglory leading to murder."

Maxims

Cases are made by circumstances: they are identified by maxims. Maxims are the common coin of moral discourse: passed back and forth, rubbed smooth and often highly inflated. They are innumerable, unsystematic, often contradictory. They range from the platitudes of Polonius's advice, "Neither borrower nor lender be" and "To thy own self be true," through the solid commonplaces of morality, such as "Do not torture innocent persons" and "To each according to his due," to ethical folk wisdom, like "don't kick a man when he's down" and "one favor deserves another." Casuists allude, explicitly or implicitly, to the maxims which appear, almost spontaneously, in any case. They organize their cases usually around the revered maxims of the Judeo-Christian Decalogue.

There are maxims aplenty in the case of the contemned captain. One should not pursue in vengeance, says Escobar, echoing a scriptural maxim frequently quoted by casuists in self defense cases. "Vegeance is mine, sayeth the Lord." A utilitarian maxim underlies the proviso, "avoid murders harmful to society." The many maxims embedded in the paradigmatic self defense argument underlie this case. The self defense argument stated most lucidly by Thomas Aquinas was woven out of several important maxims of great strength, both taken from Roman juris- prudence and repeated in canon law: "force may be repelled by force" and "response to force must be within the limits of a blameless defense." As the casuists debate this case, they ask whether the maxims which, on the face of it, might be invoked to condemn or justify, really do fit the circumstances. It finally comes clear to them that one of the key maxims of the self defense paradigm does not at all fit the case, namely, the limits of a blameless defense. The case of the insulted captain, then, is finally read out of the analogies which can plausibly follow from the paradigm.

It is important to note that casuists never attempt to systematize maxims: they do not use them as axioms to construct an argument; they do not marshal them into lexical orderings; they do not even worry much about "justifying them." They simply invoke them, much as ordinary folk do in arguing moral matters. Their primary concern is whether this maxim "fits" these circumstances.

This unsystematized and uncritical use of the maxims of common morality may be a strength or a weakness of casuistry: this we can leave to discussion. But it certainly refutes a misunderstanding of classical casuistry. A remark of Dan Callahan's expresses this misunderstanding: he speaks of "Roman Catholic moral theology as an essentially deductive kind (of system), with well-established primary principles and a . . . highly refined casuistical thinking."[25] Casuistry is not deduc- tive; it really isn't a system. It is an art or, more properly, it is an exercise of practical wisdom, in the Aristotelian sense, or of the virtue of prudence, in the Thomistic tradition. Casuists did, indeed, know and love the natural law doctrine, but they did not see it as "an essentially deductive system." The primary paradigm of self defense, as expressed by Aquinas, does indeed make a natural law reference, "it is natural for a being to seek to preserve itself in being as far as it can," but this "primary precept of natural law," as he calls it, is not used as an axiomatic principle of deductive reasoning.[16]

An Arguable Case

This leads me to a feature of casuistry which is of crucial importance. Casuists were accustomed to attach to their case what was called "a note." This was a statement of their estima- tion of the strength of the case and of the measure of confidence the reader could have in the opinion. The note was often mad- deningly brief: it would say, "certain," "more probable," "prob- ably," "less probable." But behind that brief note raged the most vigorous battle of casuistry: how to determine certainty in moral matters. The controversy is too complex to retell here.[17] However, it is enough to see it in order to recognize how far casuistry is from a deductive system: its aim was not to lead the mind, through ineluctable steps of formal argument, to a compelling truth, but to reveal, by juxtaposition of maxims and circumstance, an opinion which could be reasonably entertained. It occasionally noted certainty, as in the primary paradigms, but for the most part it noted that a case was more convincing or less convincing (our translation of the casuists' "probabilior or minus probabilis").

For most of its history, the case of the contemned captain never merited more than a note of "probabilis," which we would translate, "arguable." This is not much of a commendation in a moral argument. As the connection between life, goods and honor weakened in the casuists' minds, it became "theoretically arguable, but certainly not to be put into practice," a somewhat tortuous note which one great casuist, Lugo, said was rather silly, for ethical opinions are entertained only with a view to practice. Finally, long after the argument had petered out, an exasperated casuist devised a note that reflected the final word on the case, "bloody, vain, fleeting, fictitious and to be despised by every Christian."[18]

The plausibility of argument reveals another essential feature of casuistry. Its structure is not that of formal logical argument but of rhetoric. "Aha," the reader will say, "I always thought so: this isn't philosophy at all, but more clever elocution." "Rhetorical" and "casuistical" are indeed synonyms. But wait: I speak of rhetoric respectfully. Until almost this century, it was an esteemed discipline, concerned with the construction of argument about the contingent and the probable. Its aim is persuasion: not to be understood as swaying gullible minds by specious reasons, but leading reflective minds to reasonable opinions about those things which, by their nature, cannot be demonstrated formally. It is the structure of rhetorical argument, rather than its stylistic devices, that we believe appropriate for casuistry. This structure reveals the various ways in which claims can be supported by grounds, i.e., facts, opinions; how convincingly, plausibly, presumably, these claims can be asserted; and how they can be overturned by rebuttals and limited by exceptions.[19] This admittedly untidy form of presentation is very much at home in casuistry, but quite distasteful to philosophy which will be seized with a passion to clean it up. How often one hears the ethicist tell the perplexed: "your reasoning about this case needs to be clarified," i.e., set out in logical form and fitted into a system whereby conclusions can be inferred from principles. Casuistry, perhaps to its detriment, but, we think, to its merit, does not make this offer. In this lies its major distinction from modern moral philosophy. In this appears its baroque exuberance, its luxury of detail in contrast to the rigid clean lines of the Bauhaus logical, systematic reconstruction of morality.

Resolution

Classical casuistry was eminently practical. Its aim was not only to understand a moral problem but to resolve it. The casuists usually ended their discussion of a case with the phrase, "unde resolves." This can be translated, "Thus, you may conclude." But this translation, while correct, misses the flavor of the Latin "resolves." Its basic meaning is "to loosen, to untie," and, when used by the casuists, echos the scriptural text invoked by the Church as its license for sacramental confession, "What you loose (solveritis) on earth, shall be loosed in heaven" (Matthew 18.18). Casuistry aimed at informing persons that their conscience was not bound by a prohibition and that they could act or had acted "in good conscience."

A modern casuistry issues in a resolution of a case, not in the sense of a final, certain answer, but as a recommendation. The recommendation or counsel arrives from the perception that the relevant maxims fit the circumstances perfectly, adequately or barely. The resolution is offered as certain or plausible or arguable. This is obviously not a "conclusion" (literally a "closing" of the case) as is the final judgment of a deductively valid syllogism. Few moral cases, apart from the primary paradigms, are "conclusive." Rather, in accord with the casuistic approach, it is a thoughtful word of advice that this way to proceed does or does not seem to comport with reflective assessment of maxim and circumstances.

The casuist and the moral philosopher will differ greatly on this point. The moral philosopher will often warn the audience, "I do not presume to deliver an answer; I merely examine the process of thought whereby **you** might seek your own answer." The casuist would say, "You must, of course, make your own decision, but I can offer you a resolution to the problem which others, on due examination, have found reasonable. If your case is the same or closely analogous, this resolution is likely to be the best one."

Behind this approach lies a vast field of moral epistemology: the relation of knowledge to action. Most of the great moral philosophers have explored it but it still has unmapped areas. A serious attempt to do casuistry might inspire new inquiries, a proper task of moral theory. But, the resolution of particular moral questions cannot await a finely detailed cartography of moral psychology. Advice can and must be offered.

Conclusion

Permit me to refer again, with due modesty, to the volume, CLINICAL ETHICS. It is a casuistical book. Like many other bioethics books, it has many cases. But unlike these others, it offers no ethical theory. Its four chapters are organized, not around ethical principles, like Benevolence and Respect for Autonomy, nor around topics which can be analyzed rhetorically, such as abortion and euthanasia, but around the clusters of factual circumstances more relevant to medical decisions: medical indications, preferences, quality of life and external factors, such as costs, scarcity of resources. Each chapter refers to many maxims, from "do no harm" to "greater good of greater number." What makes the book casuistic is that the circumstances and the maxims are examined in paradigm and analogous cases with a view toward a resolution noted as plausible, arguable, obligatory, or permissible. It offers counsel about the action or policy which best fits in these or analogous circumstances. Those who read it will agree with many, doubt some, and disagree with certain resolutions, for which they will offer resolutions more fitting to the case.

I'm sure that some readers are stunned. I appear to have espoused confusion over clarity, rhetoric over logic, opinion over certainty. I have succumbed to the most unrestrained relativism and so confirmed your worst suspicions about casuistry. All this is the matter of debate. In anticipation of that debate, allow me several final comments.

First, it should be apparent that Toulmin and I do not believe that casuistry is **applied ethics**, at least not in the sense that cases are resolved by application, through operations of formal logic, of an ethical theory, be it utilitarian, contractarian, or whatever. Ethics can use cases, didactically or dialectically, to show how its manner of reasoning is to be carried out. Casuistry does not **use** cases: it **has** cases and seeks to aid in their resolution by pointing, through paradigm and analogy, to the more or less arguable fit of moral maxims in particular circumstances. It has to take the cases that come to it, whether or not they are convenient illustrations of a system. A remark of R. M. Hare reveals the difference between moral philosophy and casuistry:

> When we are doing the selection [of general principles] we ought not to pay too much attention to particular cases, actual or hypothetical, which are not at all usual or are likely to reoccur. For we are selecting our principles as practical guides in the world as it really is and not as it would be

if composed of incidents out of short
stories.[20]

Casuistry is constantly being offered the unusual and the
unlikely case. It undertakes, perhaps too boldly, to resolve
them for what they are rather than what they would be within a
system of axiomatic principles.

We must recall that the pioneer of bioethics, Joseph
Fletcher, was an avowed situationist, a position quite close to
casuistry.[21] His casuistry appealed greatly to his medical
audience, which recognized in it the doctor's maxim, "each case
is different." At the same time, his casuistry came under fire,
from theologians and philosophers, who excoriated him as an
unprincipled relativist. Fletcher, casuist in spirit, was not,
in my opinion, sufficiently casuist in method. He lacks the
strong appreciation of paradigm and analogy: all his cases are
too much on a par. He swallows up the multiplicity of maxims in
a major maxim, "love one another," and thus tends to obscure the
circumstantial power of individual maxims which have little to do
with love, such as "force may be repelled by force." Nevertheless, it might have been more advantageous for the identity and
mission of bioethics had it stayed with and strengthened its
casuistic origins instead of seeking a spurious certitude in
ethical theory.

Finally, a word of defense for my antique example, the case
of the contemned captain. In itself, it is a mere historical
oddity. But the pattern of casuistic argument which surrounded
it is strikingly contemporary. Our current bioethical discussions about killing and letting die arise from the primary
paradigms of self defense which, as the casuist knew, contain
crucial distinctions about intentions and effects of action.
While not relevant to the case of the contemned captain, the
distinction between "acting" and "refraining" is also a casuistic
distinction which appears in the treatise on the Fifth Commandment. An interesting example of the difference between the moral
philosopher's and the casuist's approach to this distinction can
be found in the exchange between Bruce Russell, Richard Trammell
and Paul Menzel in the JOURNAL OF MEDICINE AND PHILOSOPHY.[22]
Russell and Trammell approach the question in the style of modern
moral philosophy; Menzel comes as close as a moral philosopher
can come to the casuistic approach: fitting the distinction (the
maxim) to different types of cases with greater or less
suitability.

Finally, our current political debates about nuclear
armaments turn on the maxim upon which the casuists relied to
resolve the case of the contemned captain, defense moderated by
need for self preservation: a condition which, it appears,
nuclear warfare cannot meet. It has moved too far from the

126

primary paradigm to be an arguable analogy and, like Concina's note to the case of the insulted captain, is "bloody, vain, foolish and despicable to all reasonable persons."

FOOTNOTES

[1] Arthur Caplan, "Teaching Medical Ethics in the Clinical Setting. Applying Morality to Advances in Biomedicine," in NEW KNOWLEDGE IN THE BIOMEDICAL SCIENCES, ed. W. Bondeson, T. Engelhardt, Jr., S. Spicker and J. White (Dordecht: Reidel, 1982).

[2] Kai Nielsen, "On Being Skeptical About Applied Ethics," this volume, pp. 93-113

[3] Terrence F. Ackerman, "What Bioethics Should Be," JOURNAL OF MEDICINE AND PHILOSOPHY, 5(1980), pp. 260-275.

[4] J. Glover, "It Makes No Difference Whether I Do It or Not," PROCEEDINGS OF ARISTOTELEAN SOCIETY, Supp.Vol. 49 (1975), p. 183.

[5] Baruch Spinoza, ETHICS, ed. J. Gutmann, (New York: Harner, 1949).

[6] Albert Jonsen, "Can an Ethicist be a Consultant?," in FRONTIERS IN MEDICAL ETHICS, ed. Virginia Abernethy (Cambridge, Mass.: Ballinger, 1980), pp. 157-171. Almost no scholarly studies of classical casuistry exist. The articles on "Casuistry" in the NEW CATHOLIC ENCYCLOPEDIA (New York: McGraw-Hill, 1967) and in the DICTIONARY OF THE HISTORY OF IDEAS (New York: Scribners, 1968) are introductory. Bishop Kenneth Kirk's CONSCIENCE AND ITS PROBLEMS (London: Longmans Green, 1927) is a modern example of classical casuistry in the Anglican tradition.

[7] Henry Sidgwick, OUTLINES OF THE HISTORY OF ETHICS (Boston: Beacon Press, 1961), p. 153.

[8] Paul Ramsey, THE PATIENT AS PERSON (New Haven: Yale University Press, 1970), p. xviii.

[9] Blaise Pascal, THE PROVINCIAL LETTERS, ed. A. Krailsheimer (Baltimore: Penguin Books, 1967) Letter XI, p. 170.

[10] Albert Jonsen, Mark Siegler and William Winslade, CLINICAL ETHICS (New York: Macmillan, 1982).

[11] Stephen Toulmin, "Ethics and Equity: The Tyranny of Principles," HASTINGS CENTER REPORT, 11(1982), pp. 31-39.

[12] A. Escobar, LIBER THEOLOGIAE MORALIS LYONS, 1644, Tr. I., ex. 7, n. 48; cited in Pascal, op. cit., Letter VII, p. 170.

[13]Thomas Aquinas, COMMENTARY ON THE SENTENCES OF PETER LOMBARD IV, d. 33, q. 1, a.1.

[14]IV Council of the Laterna (1215). H. Denzinger, ENCHIRIDION SYMBOLORUM. (Fribourg: Herder, 1965), n. 812; D. Robertson, "A Note on the Classical Origin of Circumstances," STUDIES IN PHILOLOGY 13(1946), pp. 6-14.

[15]Daniel Callahan, "Bioethics as a Discipline," HASTINGS CENTER REPORT1(Feb. 1973), p. 72.

[16]Aquinas, SUMMA THEOLOGIAE I-II, q. 64, a. 7.

[17]THE NEW CATHOLIC ENCYCLOPEDIA, "Morality, Systems of," (New York: McGraw-Hill, 1967), V. 9, p. 1131.

[18]D. Concina, THEOLOGIA CHRISTIANA DOGMATICO-MORALIS, Naples, 1772. Book VII, Ch. 5, p. 237.

[19]S. Toulmin, R. Rieke and A. Janik, AN INTRODUCTION TO REASONING (New York: Macmillan, 1979); S. Toulmin, THE USES OF ARGUMENT (Cambridge: Cambridge University Press, 1958), ch. 3.

[20]R. M. Hare, "Can the Moral Philosopher Help?" in PHILOSOPHICAL MEDICAL ETHICS: ITS NATURE AND SIGNIFICANCE, ed. H. Tristram Engelhardt, Jr. and Stuart Spicker (Dordecht: Reidel, 1977), p. 59.

[21]Joseph Fletcher, MORALS AND MEDICINE (Boston: Beacon Press, 1954); and SITUATION ETHICS (Philadelphia: Westminster Press, 1966).

[22]B. Russell, "On the Presumption Against Taking Life"; R. Trammell, "On the Nonequivalency of Saving Life and Not Taking Life"; and P. Menzel, "Are Killing and Letting Die Morally Different in Medical Contexts?" JOURNAL OF MEDICINE AND PHILOSOPHY 4(1979), pp. 244-294.

CAN APPLIED ETHICS BE EFFECTIVE IN HEALTH CARE AND SHOULD IT STRIVE TO BE?*[1]

Arthur L. Caplan

I. MORAL EFFICACY IN MEDICINE

A number of philosophers, theologians, and others with a major interest in ethics have, in recent times, found themselves plying their trades in the confines of a hospital or medical center. The extent of their involvement has grown to proportions which are sufficient to permit an inquiry into what exactly it is that these persons are supposed to be doing in such settings. This inquiry leads inevitably to a further and more significant question: are philosophers and others engaged in what has come to be called "applied ethics" in the "real world" of medicine able to do anything useful there? In mulling over such questions, it may be useful for the reader to ponder two examples which stand out in my own mind as the occasions upon which, through my involvement in a medical center, I felt I was most effective with reference to matters of applied ethics.

The first incident occurred in the course of teaching in the hospital of a large urban medical center. The elective was entitled "Ethics Rounds" and was team taught with a psychiatrist and an internist. The course consisted of visiting various patients selected by students, interviewing the patients, and discussing some of the moral issues that the students and teachers felt were raised by the cases.

Early on in the course the students had selected a 90-year-old woman with a fractured arm for an interview. She had no relatives, and the students were worried about what might happen to her upon discharge from the hospital. I came to the class fully prepared to discourse on theories of distributive justice at a moment's notice, since I rather naively believed the students might benefit greatly from a disquisition on Mill, Rawls, and Nozick in trying to figure out what to do with the old woman.

As soon as the medical instructors and students had gathered together, we hurriedly set off to find and interview the old woman. We all burst into her room just as she was in the process of defecating. To my surprise, no one was deterred by her

*I would like to acknowledge the support of the National Endowment for the Humanities and the Carnegie Corporation of New York in the preparation of this paper. I am grateful to my colleagues at the Hastings Center for numerous spirited discussions of many of the issues raised in the paper.

behavior, and both the psychiatrist and the internist proceeded immediately to interview the woman about her life plans, goals, and personal aspirations. I remained uncharacteristically silent during this exchange, and it was only when the class had returned to the confines of the psychiatry lounge to discuss the case that I proffered the opinion that it might have been better to wait until the woman had finished her excretory functions before interviewing her. This observation was greeted with some consternation by both students and other teachers. Of course I was correct, they conceded. Privacy was important to patients, as my comment showed, and physicians should not allow the press of their own busy schedules to override a patient's need for a certain amount of privacy. My insight was acknowledged with a great degree of gravity, and my esteem among the members of the course was assured for the duration of that particular clinical rotation.

The other paradigmatic example of my moral efficacy in a hospital setting resulted from a suggestion I made concerning a problem of scarce medical resources. Every summer the emergency room of the hospital filled up with persons suffering from emphysema and other respiratory ailments. The hot weather made it very difficult for such persons to breathe comfortably, and they came to the emergency room to receive oxygen. Unfortunately, there were only two oxygen units available, and there were often a dozen or more persons seeking to use them at various times during the day and night. The staff of the emergency room asked my help in developing a set of criteria for deciding what would be a fair and equitable allocation of their scarce medical resources.

My first response upon hearing their request was to consult the diverse anthologies in existence on medical ethics to see what various philosophers and theologians had to say about issues of micro-allocation and ethics. I found they had the predictable things to say about such matters -- some defended a criterion of merit, some a criterion of need, some a criterion of social utility, and some a random lottery. I was fortunately bright enough to suspect that the medical staff could have gotten that far without me or the anthology. But, in thinking about the matter further, it occurred to me that it might be possible to solve the allocation problem by ameliorating the source of the scarcity. I asked some of the emergency room staff if Medicaid/Medicare covered the provision of air conditioners in the homes of persons suffering from respiratory ailments. It turned out, much to everyone's surprise, that the machines could be prescribed and the cost reimbursed. I ascended to the status of moral guru in the emergency room, famous as the man who had solved the oxygen machine crunch.

I mention these incidents not to impress anyone with my problem-solving skills. Indeed, I believe any person of reasonable intelligence possessing a bit of perspective on the behavior of the health-care professional involved in both of these cases could have arrived at the exact same recommendations and solutions. It is interesting to note, however, that these two cases of efficacious moral action were hardly dependent on analytical rigor or theoretical moral sophistication for their genesis. Indeed, in both cases, ethical theory would have been the wrong place to turn for a solution to the issues under consideration.

II. WHAT EXACTLY IS IT THAT THOSE IN APPLIED ETHICS DO?

Of course it ought to be noted that philosophers and others working in medical settings engage in other activities besides behavioral reform. Philosophers with a background in ethics teach in various types of settings; attend rounds; serve on various kinds of committees, such as Institutional Review Boards and hospital 'ethics' committees; engage in health-policy formulation at the federal, state, and local levels; offer consultation and advice to interested parties in hospitals about a wide variety of ethical matters; and, on occasion, serve as moral fire fighters, rushing to various places within the hospital to help solve a moral dilemma or resolve a staff dispute. Not all philosophers working in medical centers do all of these things, but many of them have at one time or another been asked to serve as a teacher, lay representative, advisor, policymaker, or arbitrator. There are even media reports of philosophers and theologians prowling the floors of some hospitals armed with an electronic beeper and clad in a white coat, the better to respond efficaciously to moral crises and ethical emergencies.

"Beeper ethics" aside, it seems that philosophers and other persons with expertise in ethics believe that there are all sorts of contributions that they can and should make to the operation of medical centers and the wellbeing of staff and patients. What is less evident in considering these activities is exactly what skills and what expertise those in applied ethics think they possess that would make them effective in any way with regard to some or all of the various roles health professionals ask them to assume.

III. PHILOSOPHICAL QUALIFICATIONS FOR MEDICAL EMPLOYMENT

One skill that philosophers seem to pride themselves on, in particular, is that of conceptual analysis. Oftentimes in the course of trying to explain to the uninitiated of health care what it is that philosophers do, those in philosophy and, in particular, applied ethics will mention such talents as being able to analyze the meanings of words, detect logical confusions and fallacies, and the ability to establish canons of sound and valid argumentation. Thus, one skill that someone expert in applied ethics can provide to those working in a medical setting is felt to be that of patrolling and policing logical malefactors.

Second, many persons working in applied ethics believe themselves to be in possession of a body or corpus of knowledge concerning ethical theories which can be brought to bear on moral problems arising in the practice of medicine. This knowledge includes both a mastery of ethical traditions within philosophy and, perhaps, theology, and an understanding of the ways in which moral beliefs and opinions can legitimately be justified through linking them to appropriate moral theories drawn from these traditions. Just as an engineer utilizes his or her understanding of the theories of physics to solve practical problems of transportation or heating of the sort which arise in everyday life, so the applied ethicist working in a medical setting can bring to bear the theoretical insights and lemmas of contemporary moral theory to solve the everyday moral quandaries of hospital life.

Third, some philosophers and ethical experts have noted that they bring an especially rare commodity into the health-care setting, the skill or ability to remain disinterested and neutral about moral events of the sort that arise in medicine. Philosophers who work in medical settings often view themselves as impartial observers of the medical scene. They are persons without a vested interest in the kinds of care that are delivered, the safety and efficacy of particular procedures, and they do not have a political need to align themselves with any individual or group within the medical settings. This perspective allows them, so they believe, to weigh alternatives and reflect upon policies in ways that those caught up in the system, either as providers or recipients of health care, cannot. Thus, as the two vignettes given earlier suggest, impartiality permits a person engaged in applied ethics to see the medical world in ways that are not available to those who are part of the scenery, often with beneficial consequences for all.

IV. THE "ENGINEERING MODEL" OF APPLIED ETHICS

This picture of ethics, emphasizing conceptual clarification, mastery of ethical theory, and impartiality, can usefully be referred to as the "engineering model" of applied ethics. It presumes that: (1) there is a body of knowledge concerning ethics that persons can be more or less knowledgeable about; (2) this knowledge becomes "applied" in medical settings by: (a) deducing conclusions from theories in light of relevant empirical facts and descriptions of circumstances and (b) analyzing properly the process of the deduction (i.e., watching for logical fallacies, ambiguities in the meaning of key terms, improper classifications of entities, misdescriptions, etc.); and (3) the process of applying ethical knowledge to moral problems in medicine can and must be carried out in an impartial, disinterested, value-free manner.

It is interesting to note that the engineering model is quite analogous to the model of nomological explanation regnant for so many years in the philosophy of the natural and social sciences. Explanation on the old N-D model was held simply to be a matter of deduction from theory, the deduction being accomplished by the supplementation of laws and principles with the appropriate initial and boundary conditions, bridge principles, and empirical descriptions. The process of explanation was to be carried out in a value-free way by impartial souls dedicated solely to the advancement of human understanding and scientific progress.

In its applied ethics reincarnation, moral justification has assumed the role of explanation. The process of explaining by subsuming data under a set of theoretical principles is directly mimicked by viewing the subsumption of moral "data" under a set of hierarchically ordered moral principles as the key to justification. Impartiality is the ethos held to pervade both undertakings. Why this model has taken hold in ethics when it has undergone such drastic revisions and modifications in the philosophy of science is surely an intellectual issue worthy of serious examination. But what is perhaps more interesting is the degree to which those who do applied work in ethics are wedded to the engineering model as a matter of self-perception, both of what it is they do and how it is they ought do it.

V. HAVE PHILOSOPHERS AND OTHERS OPERATING WITH THE ENGINEERING MODEL BEEN EFFECTIVE IN MEDICINE?

There are numerous and obvious reasons for doubting whether it is possible to show if medical ethics, as practiced by on-site medical ethicists, has made any difference to the practice of medicine. Medicine is hardly an isolated system and, whatever one thinks of the appropriateness of doing beeper ethics, those philosophers in the trade have not been prowling hospital corridors for all that long a period of time.

Nevertheless, a few general observations about efficacy can be made. On the whole, those doing applied ethics have been far more effective in influencing the formulation of health policy at the federal level than at the bedside. Philosophers, both through arguments in the literature and through direct participation in the policy process, have had a hand in bringing about the creation and maintenance of committees, review procedures, regulations, and institutional controls pertaining to the practice of medicine and the delivery of health care. In large measure, for example, the continued existence of a system of Institutional

135

Review Boards at all medical centers receiving research monies
from the National Institutes of Health can be traced directly to
recent moral concerns about human experimentation and the atten-
dant ethical issues this raises. These issues were and continue
to be presented to a wide public audience by persons doing
applied ethics.

Those in the applied ethics trade have been far less
successful at some of the other roles and activities they have
been asked or assigned, or have volunteered, to undertake. The
teaching of medical ethics in the medical school curriculum has
not been received with a great deal of enthusiasm by its intended
audience. Students and faculty often find ethics courses boring
and irrelevant. Many assign them low priority vis-a-vis other
subjects. The ground swell of interest that surrounded the introduction of the subject in medical schools seems to have peaked,
and there is some evidence that certain schools have, as often
happens with rapid innovations in the medical curriculum, tired
of this particular subject and may be moving on to newer and more
lucrative ones.

Similarly, poor grades can be given in assessing the ability
of philosophers and others in applied ethics to work well with
medical personnel on matters of morality. Many in applied ethics
simply find clinical work uncomfortable and do not choose to do
it. When they do do it, however, health-care personnel often
find themselves highly frustrated with the end results. As one
clinician acquaintance of mine observed about philosophers-in-
residence in medical settings, "You guys like to talk about
ethics, but you don't want to do any ethics." Health-care
practitioners expect practical advice and counsel about actions
they should take regarding specific patients. When such advice
is not forthcoming, they become frustrated with the logic chop-
ping of applied ethicists and turn to each other (or, rather,
return to each other) for moral guidance and psychological
support.

Few philosophers have been asked to help formulate sensitive
hospital policies such as those governing admission to neonatal
intensive care units or discharge from intensive care units. The
issues of allocation and equity which arise on a daily basis in
medical practice are usually resolved by senior medical personnel
behind doors firmly closed to the wisdom of moral philosophers.

Those philosophers and theologians who are asked to "para-
chute" in to solve various crisis situations, such as when
doctors and nurses are at odds about various hospital practices
or when physical therapists, social workers, and occupational
therapists are engaged in battles over turf, professional responsibility, or professional ego, do not last long. They usually
meet the same fate as the psychiatrists who are likely to have

preceded them -- interest if they take sides, polite universal
hostility if they do not.

Overall, the record of efficacy is a mixed bag. There have
been some real policy triumphs at the national level; some
schools have found philosophers to be useful in the classroom or
on regulatory committees; and many health-care practitioners pay
more attention to moral issues than they did before the applied
ethicist appeared. On the other hand, most health practitioners
find the writing and teaching of those in applied ethics hopelessly opaque and irrelevant, student interest in courses is
weak, medical personnel find the skills of conceptual clarification and logical analysis to be of little use, and few philosophers have been asked to become involved in an active, ongoing
way in hospital policy formulation on a day-to-day basis.

VI. WHY HAS APPLIED ETHICS ENJOYED A MIXED RECORD OF SUCCESS IN
     MEDICINE?

If it is true that those doing applied ethics have not, to
date, succeeded in carrying out the various kinds of tasks they
find themselves engaged in within medical settings, then why
might this be so? There is a temptation to turn, in light of the
engineering model, to ethical theory as the cause of any failures
that exist. Perhaps current moral theory is not adequate for
solving the kinds of problems that exist in contemporary medicine.
Ethics, like sociology and the other social sciences, must await
its Newton, if those doing applied ethics are to be properly
armed with theories that would enable them to work effectively
with medical practitioners in solving the everyday moral puzzles
of hospital life.

It may be true that some of the failures and disappointments
arising in the course of recent work in applied ethics in medical
centers can be blamed on inadequate theories in ethics proper.
However, it may be that some of the difficulties have more to do
with the uses to which such theories are put than with the
adequacy or inadequacy of available moral theories, per se.

One difficulty confronting anyone attempting to utilize
extant moral theories of justice, rights, or whatever to solve
moral problems in hospital settings is that the problems are
always complex and murky, particularly as a consequence of the
dynamic nature of morality in medicine. Much of moral theory
today presumes a static system whereby the abilities, interests,
and needs of parties can be established and, once discerned,
assumed to be constant. However, in the real world of medical
morality, interests and needs constantly change and evolve.
Patients learn to adjust to illness, nurses develop dislikes for
particular patients, house staff grow eager to find an "inter-

esting case" after dealing with a run of twenty alcoholics, and so on.

Not only do the phenomena of moral life constantly change and evolve in medicine, but it is not always clear how best to describe and individuate the moral data that appear in this constantly shifting context. Just as the N-D model of explanation in the philosophy of science foundered on the shoals of the observation/theory distinction and the impossibility of locating a pure observation language, the engineering model of applied ethics shows signs of collapse when put to the test of locating pure moral "facts" whose descriptions are both intersubjectively verifiable and unbiased. Those in applied ethics have two difficulties in finding moral facts to submit to the test of moral theory. First, they are not always very good at knowing enough about medicine to understand a situation adequately and describe it. And, second, even when they do, they come to the medical setting with a vast array of sophisticated preconceptions and theoretical biases that influence their moral perceptions and classifications. This view of ethical theory presumes it is possible simply to locate moral facts and test them against theory. But the process of observation, individuation, and description is no easier in the moral realm than it is in the scientific. So simple-minded a view of the relationship between fact and theory in ethics is certain to fail to be useful for purposes of problem solving.

But the failures of applied ethics to solve all of the various problems that have been put before it cannot be attributed simply to an inadequate view of moral theory. The source of most problems for those involved in doing applied ethics is in great measure the engineering model of application which governs much of what is done with available moral theory in solving moral problems in medicine.

VII. THE INADEQUACIES OF THE ENGINEERING MODEL OF APPLIED ETHICS

There are four important ways in which the engineering model of applied ethics both minimizes the efficacious use of moral theories and hinders the utility of applied ethicists in medical settings.

Problem Selection and the Definition of Moral Problems

On the engineering model of applied ethics, application is equated with deduction from a theory. Unfortunately, such a view presupposes that the analysis of what counts as a moral problem in medicine is either self-evident or predetermined by health professionals. On this model, the health professional presents a moral problem to a person trained in the fine points of ethics, who can then proceed to grind the problem through the available

138

moral theories. While this kind of process sometimes works well in analyzing moral issues in medicine, more often than not those seeking advice or help in answering a moral problem are not in the best position to define the nature of the problem. By emphasizing deduction from theory as the main task of the applied ethicist, the engineering model obscures the fact that problem analysis and diagnosis are just as important in medical settings as is the solving of moral puzzles.

The situation confronting a person attempting to do ethics in the health-care setting is not all that dissimilar from that confronting a clinician in treating a patient with a medical complaint. Clinicians treat the complaints of patients as possible evidence of a medical problem. But they do not view what patients have to say as definitive with respect to identifying what the problem is, or even with respect to whether a problem actually exists.

Similarly, in analyzing a moral problem in medicine, it would be wrong to take the complaints of health-care professionals or patients simply at face value. Rather than attempt to solve problems within the framework of those who present them, as is encouraged on the engineering model, the applied ethicist must feel free to reinterpret complaints, disregard some issues, and, occasionally, move beyond the issues as initially framed by health-care professionals. Otherwise, applied ethics can become merely the palliative treatment of the symptomatology of ethical discontent.

Overemphasis on Means, Not Ends

Health-care professionals, like other busy people, place high value on the efficient solution of problems and quandaries. Those doing applied ethics along the lines indicated in the engineering model are highly susceptible to professional pressures on them to analyze and solve problems quickly. Efficiency becomes a prized value, while the analysis of the legitimacy of medical ends is easily discouraged. It is difficult to practice medicine and at the same time have someone around constantly questioning the value of the effort. However, after seeing case after case of 95-year-old women tied to their beds in intensive care units in order to permit the administration of drugs and fluids with a minimum amount of patient resistance, one may become convinced that there is a real need to resist the siren call of efficiency inherent in the engineering model in order to probe more deeply into the ultimate aims and goals of various medical endeavors.

Taking Medical Common Sense Seriously

There is a very strong tendency which the engineering model does nothing to discourage to view persons doing applied ethics as on a par with other consultants and experts who are present in medical settings. Just as the cardiologist and endocrinologist have their domains of expertise, so the philosopher and theologian is often thought expert in moral matters. Such a view discourages those doing applied ethics from taking seriously what health professionals have to say about moral issues in medicine. More important, it discourages close attention to the realities of illness and anxiety for patients and their families. By locating moral competence in the applied ethicist, the engineering model discounts the realities -- of the sick role, of the inability to cope with fear, of the experience of pain, and so on -- that are so important in understanding moral issues in medicine. All one need do is to take a casual glance through the literature on autonomy, paternalism, and personal responsibility in the journals of applied ethics to see how far moral expertise has wandered from moral reality.

Who Wants Moral Expertise and Who Can Pay for It?

Another problem inherent in the engineering model of applied ethics is that, by leaving problem definition in the hands of health professionals, the model tends to limit contacts between applied ethicists and health professionals to those health professionals who ask for help. For a variety of reasons, those likely to ask for help are physicians. This means that the tendency is to focus on moral dilemmas faced by physicians in clinical settings, and for those doing applied ethics to be identified with physicians. The fact that physicians usually are also the ones most often in the position of paying for the presence of persons doing applied ethics in medical settings does little to encourage attention to other parties. The engineering model not only skews ethics in the direction of technical competence, but also limits philosophical attention to those who seek and can pay for technical assistance.

VIII. WHEN FAILURE IS NOT FAILURE

There are a variety of reasons for suspecting that some of the difficulties encountered by those doing applied ethics in medical centers can be traced back to inadequacies in both current moral theories and in the model of application dominant in applied ethics today. But it ought to be noted that, while the engineering model assumes that those who ask for help or seek aid are sincere in doing so, this is not always the case. Sincerity is no more to be taken for granted in dealing with medical professionals than it is with persons claiming to want help in any walk of life.

There are a number of reasons why health professionals may want to involve applied ethicists in their work that have nothing whatsoever to do with resolving problems or grounding moral beliefs on a firmer analytical foundation.

Moral Theorizing as Diversionary

There are all sorts of ways in which labeling a problem as a moral issue can be useful in diverting attention from other types of problems that arise in medical settings. Thus, for example, it is far better, from the point of view of the hospital administration, to have nurses discussing the morality of strikes than it is to have them engaging in such activities. If one must have a public participant on an Institutional Review Board panel for reviewing human subjects research, it is much easier to deal with an academic than a real, live resident from the immediate hospital neighborhood. It is far easier to begin a moral discussion about the allocation of scarce resources, such as kidney dialysis units, than to ask health practitioners and patients to live with the fact that society has decided not to fund a sufficient number of machines to treat all who are in need.

Applied Ethics as Cooptative

Administrators and department chairs are frequently confronted with protests and complaints from underlings about the operation of a floor, unit, or ward. The usual response of medical administrators to such crisis situations is to find a way for staff to "let off some steam." People faced with a crisis are often quite prepared to utilize applied ethicists as harmless targets for the venting of anger and rage by hospital staff. However, often the complaints of the staff are legitimate and the invoking of ethics and moral analysis serves merely to sidetrack legitimate complaints and grievances that should be directed elsewhere.

Moral Engineering as Ceremony

Procrastination is a marvelous response to crises of all sorts, and this strategy has its proponents in health care as well. Oftentimes someone seeking the guidance of a moral guru is more interested in appearance than solutions. The time-consuming ethical meanderings of a verbose moral philosopher can provide a concrete and lengthy demonstration of concern over some thorny moral issue. Health-care professionals enjoy a performance as much as anyone else, and the virtuosity of moral engineers, while it is rarely taken seriously, can be at least temporarily entertaining for all concerned.

IX. THE ART OF MORAL ENGINEERING

I have been fairly harsh on the engineering model of applied ethics in this essay. However, I am very much aware of the fact that engineering is a valuable and helpful activity even in a field such as ethics. But those who do applied ethics in any field must be aware of the limits and dangers inherent in the engineering model. In the rush to be efficacious, it would be a grave mistake to lose the freedom and independence requisite for sound prescriptive inquiry into any ethical issue.

Those who engage in applied ethics must decide for themselves exactly when and for whom ethical engineering is appropriate. In assessing the fruits of their labors, they must also remain aware that there are numerous reasons why efforts by applied ethicists in medical settings fail. Not all invitations to help are authentic, and there are many circumstances in which the process of doing ethics is more highly prized than the results of such a process. It is also true that certain moral dilemmas which chronically arise in medical settings serve various sorts of adaptive functions for health professionals. The prospect of finally resolving such dilemmas can be far more frightening to the persons involved than the need to accommodate their existence.

Ethical engineering like other forms of engineering is an art. It requires practical knowledge, theoretical understanding, and experience. It also requires a certain amount of independence and tolerance from those who engage the engineer. After all, moral efficacy is desirable only when the right questions are being addressed.

FOOTNOTES

[1]Reprinted from ETHICS 93 (January 1983), pp. 311-319, with permission of The University of Chicago Press.

MEDICAL ETHICS IN THE CLINICAL SETTING:
A CRITICAL REVIEW OF ITS CONSULTATIVE, PEDAGOGICAL
AND INVESTIGATIVE METHODS

Terrence F. Ackerman

Introduction

As a component in American medical education, medical ethics faces the joys and tribulations of a budding adolescence. Its joys are newfound opportunities. Before the late sixties, no formal programs in medical ethics or medical humanities existed in American medical schools. By contrast, a recent survey indicates that at least sixty medical colleges now have some formal humanities component in the curriculum.[1] Better than a dozen programs have two or more full-time faculty members who teach in the medical humanities. Moreover, informal descriptions indicate that, in at least four programs, faculty members carry on a regular schedule of clinical activities, including participation in teaching rounds and grand rounds, presentation of clinical case conferences, and consultation on individual patient care decisions.

But the opportunities have generated some typical dilemmas of adolescence. There is the intense "peer pressure." Placed in an environment quite different from the liberal arts curriculum, medical ethics programs face the challenge of developing teaching activities which dovetail with the settings, methods and practical objectives of medical education. Moreover, medical ethics is struggling to define the appropriate limits of its independence from the parent disciplines which spawned its inquiries, such as philosophy and religious studies. In doing so, it is compelled to examine how the focus, methods and style of its scholarly research must reflect and differ from these parent disciplines in meeting the needs of medical education and practice. Most importantly, though, medical ethics is in search of its "identity" as a **bona fide** component of medical education: a clear conception of its purpose, a clarification of the roles in which medical ethicists might fulfill this function, and an understanding of the methods appropriate to both the diverse roles and underlying purpose. My remarks are intended to facilitate this passage of medical ethics into secure adult identity as a field of scholarly endeavor.

It is a commonplace that practice precedes reflection but cannot long persist without it. Situations arise whose significance for practice is obscure, and inquiry is evoked to establish their import for further activities. Medical ethics utilizes the methodological tools of ethical inquiry to examine medical situations whose moral significance is unclear. Thus,

145

understanding medical ethics requires a clear conception of the purpose and structure of moral inquiry as a reflective enterprise. The initial section of my remarks are addressed to this subject.

The description of moral inquiry will provide a framework for investigating the methods and goals appropriate to the key activities of ethicists in medical academia. Of course, medical ethics as an academic field is not restricted to the confines of medical education. Many classes in medical ethics are taught in the undergraduate liberal arts curriculum and many scholars in the field do not conduct activities in the clinical setting. There are numerous roles in which scholars in the field broadly understood might conceivably function. These include service as patient care consultants to health professionals, as teachers, investigators, policy analysts, committee members, advisors to consumer groups, personal confidants to patients, etc. However, I will focus upon medical ethics as a component in medical education. Consequently, I restrict my discussion to the three activities of the medical ethicist which are most prominent in the clinical setting: consultation, teaching and research.

The Purpose and Structure of Moral Inquiry

Moral inquiry in the health care setting is evoked by situations whose moral significance for medical practice is obscure or uncertain. Three main features characterize these situations. First, choice of a course of action involves more than classification of a pathological condition and institution of the optimal therapy. Second, broader human values or aims, such as respect for autonomy or concern for the patient's well-being, suggest the appropriateness of different outcomes and courses of action. Finally, there is lack of social consensus concerning which values should take precedence and what pattern of social interaction should subsequently be instituted.

The purpose of moral inquiry is set by this practical and social context which generates moral predicaments. Its function is to identify plans of action for resolving moral dilemmas which are socially endorsable because in actual operation they will effectively and impartially realize the values (outcomes) which persons cherish as a result of such inquiry. In fulfilling this purpose, moral inquiry may focus upon a particular situation or a set of similar situations. The solution to a particular case is provided by a "course of action," while for a set of situations it is carried in a "policy." However, since the purpose and structure of moral inquiry does not differ according to its focus, I will use the terms "decision" or "plan of action" to refer indiscriminately to the different outcomes of moral inquiry.

There are several significant features of moral inquiry thus understood. First, moral investigation if successful does not issue in the discovery of moral claims which have validity independent of human choice. Rather, the objective of moral inquiry is a socially generated and endorsed moral decision or commitment which issues from the process of inquiry itself. Any health care practitioner who has wrestled with real-life moral dilemmas in the clinic knows that action must always go forth under conditions of existential anguish and uncertainty. This anguish is attributable to the need to make choices under complex empirical conditions. If answers independent of human choice were discoverable, certainty rather than anguish would characterize moral decisions. Such neat solutions are possessed only by those who approach moral issues with dogmatic preconceptions or who fail to understand the empirical complexities of the dilemmas. There are no "answers," only decisions whose formulation is more or less well-controlled by the pattern of moral inquiry itself.[2]

Second, moral inquiry is an inherently social process. This does not mean that we cannot deliberate privately regarding moral dilemmas. The lonely resident on "night call" can attest to this point. Rather, when engaging in moral inquiry we commit ourselves to determination of a plan of action which would meet the approval of all those who might engage in the same reflective process. Since moral problems are situations which evoke initial social disagreement, their resolution depends upon the articulation of a socially supportable decision. This feature of moral inquiry has an exact analogue in scientific investigation. Claims regarding the correlation of events in nature do not merit the status of knowledge unless different investigators following similar methodological steps produce similar results. Justified belief, whether moral or scientific, is a socially produced outcome.

Of course, we can never carry the social process of moral inquiry to its ideal limit. In stating the purpose of moral inquiry, the phrase "socially endorsable" is meant to capture this point: whatever the constraints of time and setting, in moral inquiry we commit ourselves to formulating a decision which is capable of receiving general social endorsement even if this endorsement cannot, in fact, now be sought.

Third, in formulating decisions in moral inquiry we commit ourselves to impartially consider the outcomes or values which all parties to the decision making process initially cherish. Of course, realization of different outcomes is oftentimes not empirically possible and priorities must be set. However, too much research in medical ethics is permeated by the "Either-Or" mentality -- either respect for autonomy or concern for the patient's well-being, etc. In actual circumstances, a plan of action can often be formulated that will take into account the outcomes which different parties to the inquiry consider valuable. Since we seek socially supportable decisions, the effort to find plans which satisfy different viewpoints is always primary in moral inquiry.

Fourth, moral inquiry seeks to formulate courses of conduct which in actual operation will **effectively** realize the outcomes that persons reflectively cherish. This point has crucial implications for medical ethics inquiry. On one hand, it means that the clinical circumstances in which proposed plans would take effect must be carefully investigated to determine how these plans might interact with existing conditions to achieve the outcomes we cherish. The social sciences, such as sociology and psychology, thus have an integral function to play in medical ethics inquiry. Unfortunately, volume upon volume of medical ethics "research" appears which makes no attempt to draw upon the benefits of hard-nosed social science research into the conditions and consequences of alternative value commitments we might make. If such research produces "correct" conclusions, the result is only an accidental accretion of the undertaking.

On the other hand, the search for plans which are effective in operation means that proposed plans must be treated as hypotheses. Proposals are fully endorsable only when they are subjected to test or confirmation in concrete operation. The projected outcome of acting upon suggested social commitments must be carefully compared with their actual outcome in achieving the reflective valuings of all persons. Discrepancy between projected and actual outcome would indicate a need for further revision of proposed plans or cherished outcomes.

The structure or pattern of moral inquiry is constituted by the set of analytic procedures which provide the means for achieving the objective of moral inquiry, i.e., the identification of plans of action which are effective in achieving socially endorsable outcomes or values. This pattern has several distinct components. One phase is the identification of problematic values. As defined above, a moral dilemma exists when different human values suggest conflicting courses of conduct. Clarification of the problem involves identification of the distinct values which are suggestive of different plans of resolution. In particular situations, the problematic values are the distinct consequences or outcomes which the respective parties to the debate initially believe to be worthy of consideration. In general form they are represented in what moral philosophers call "middle-level" moral principles: respect for autonomy, concern for the patient's well-being, justice, truth-telling, fairness, promise-keeping, concern for the well-being of groups of persons, etc. For example, in formulating a moral policy regarding non-therapeutic research with children, problematic values include concern for the well-being of potential subjects, respect for their wishes, commitment to the improved health of the pediatric population as a group, respect for parental authority, and a concern to treat various classes of pediatric subjects fairly **vis a vis** one another and other subject groups. This set of problematic values forms the framework from which development of policy proposals and revision of valued outcomes must proceed.

A second component is the formulation of alternative decisions or plans of action. As suggested above, these alternatives may be either courses of action for resolving a particular situation or a policy for dealing with a set of situations. Moreover, the set of alternatives may be quite limited (to resuscitate or not) or extremely complex (as in the case of policy options for the use of nontherapeutic research procedures with children). But however complex the alternatives, their formulation must always be undertaken with a view to instituting a set of valued outcomes which parties to the debate would accept upon reflection. Although usually overlooked by those who take the "Either-Or" approach to moral dilemmas, this may be an extremely creative phase of moral inquiry.[3]

A third component of moral inquiry is the comparison of alternative plans of action with respect to their ability to institute under existing empirical conditions some set of consequences which persons might cherish upon reflection. Under the exigencies of immediate circumstances, this component may be restricted to what Dewey has called "imaginative rehearsal."[4] In imaginative rehearsal, we project how alternative plans will interact with existing conditions to produce various outcomes, based upon our knowledge of the consequences of similar actions in similar past situations. However, when carried more toward its ideal limit, this component of moral inquiry involves the experimental test of plans of action to determine whether they will produce outcomes which can be socially endorsed. An obvious component of such experimental test is careful analytic observation of results.

Suppose, for example, that we are interested in determining a socially endorsable policy concerning the role of the physician in the informed consent process. The notion of respect for autonomy captures one valued outcome: the state of affairs in which patients select therapeutic options which accord with their life plans. One policy alternative involves the assignment to the physician of the role as information-provider only. In the experimental phase of moral inquiry, this policy must be compared with others in its capacity to produce autonomous patient behaviors. Analytic observation may suggest, for example, that various affective and social factors impede autonomous behavior by patients when physicians merely provide information. An alternative policy in which physicians also act to ameliorate these constraints may be found more effective in facilitating autonomous patient choice.

A fourth component of moral inquiry is the collection of relevant data, whether medical or psycho-social. Plans of action are not instituted in an empirical vacuum. Rather, they must interact with a varied pattern of existing conditions to achieve an eventual outcome. Consequently, knowledge of existing factors is integral to the pattern of inquiry which issues in operationally effective and justified moral beliefs. In the context of particular cases, the relevant empirical data obviously includes information regarding the medical and psychosocial status of the patient. But it also includes established general correlations among empirical factors. For example, levels of anxiety have been found to correlate inversely with retention of information disclosed in the consent setting. Such correlations may be useful not only in specific cases, but also in formulating general policies (such as an understanding of what we ought to accomplish in initial informed consent interviews).

It is important to avoid the notion that the various components of moral inquiry represent sequential and self-contained steps. On the contrary, the different phases of moral inquiry must be dynamically interrelated. For example, a particular set of problematic values points to a specific policy proposal. When put into operation, this proposal produces unexpected and disvalued results. Analysis of the results suggests an alternative plan of action not previously considered. Again, experimental comparison of alternative plans may indicate that some initially valued outcome is not achievable under existing clinical circumstances. Cherished outcomes must subsequently be altered or set in a different priority ranking as suggested by data regarding correlation of empirical factors, etc. Thus, clarification of problematic values, identification of alternative plans, experimental comparison of operational effectiveness, and correlation of existing empirical conditions are phases of inquiry which must develop in strictly conjugate fashion. Otherwise, moral inquiry cannot be successful in achieving effective and socially endorsed policies.

Having briefly reviewed the objective and structure of moral inquiry, we can now describe the general function of the medical ethicist in the clinical setting. This role is to facilitate the process of moral inquiry as the latter is applied to moral dilemmas which arise clinically. Facilitation of the process of moral inquiry involves executing the various component steps of moral inquiry. As described above, the process of moral inquiry is an inherently social enterprise. In facilitating this process in the clinical setting, the medical ethicist may serve in three distinct social roles: as consultant, pedagogue or investigator.

Medical Ethics Consultations

In examining the ethicist's role as consultant, three problems must be addressed. The first involves determining the party whom the ethicist serves and the source of authorization to act in this capacity. The second problem concerns the description of the services ethicists might provide as consultants. The third problem relates to the identification of various roles which might be mistakenly ascribed to or assumed by the ethicist as consultant.

Veatch notes that the ethicist might be retained by numerous agents: patient, family, health professionals in their professional capacity or as lay persons, etc. This seems substantially correct. The ethicist is a facilitator of moral inquiry, and each of these persons may face moral dilemmas. However, the manner in which we characterize the primary role of the ethicist as consultant depends upon our description of the general character of the moral dilemmas which most frequently arise in the clinical setting.

This description depends on whether the capabilities of patients as decision makers and the identification of strategies for respecting their autonomy are considered problematic factors in clinical moral dilemmas. For Veatch they are **not**. He assumes that patients have a ready-made ability to put their life plans into operation. Combining this claim with the fact that patients and health professionals may have divergent values, he concludes that the patient's choice should settle moral questions regarding therapeutic interaction. The health professional's role is only to provide technically competent services within the value framework set by the patient.[5]

These same assumptions also settle the role of the ethicist:

> Having said this, it seems that the obvious
> role for the clinical medical ethicist is as
> an agent for the patient. The patient, or
> the lay agent for the patient, should be
> presumed to be the primary decision maker for
> his or her own case. This should especially
> be the case when the decision involves
> ethical or related value choices.[6]

Since clinical moral dilemmas are to be resolved by the patient, the ethicist functions as a value advisor to the patient, authorized through a contractual agreement with the latter to perform specified services.

Unfortunately, this account is based upon a seriously inaccurate description of the characteristic features of moral problems which arise in the clinical setting. The extent of cognitive, affective and social constraints upon the patient's decision making is typically a key problematic factor. This, in turn, renders problematic the manner in which the health professional should interact with the patient in respecting the latter's autonomy. Whether the issue be refusal of treatment, truthtelling, discontinuation of life-prolonging therapy, involuntary commitment or numerous other dilemmas, the status of the patient as autonomous and the implications for therapeutic interaction are crucial problems.[7] This is not to deny that the best resolution of these dilemmas may sometimes involve (with Veatch) a "presumption" that the patient's choices should be accepted at face value. Rather, it is to point out that clinical situations create moral problems because conditions exist which require that this presumption be examined. Moreover, this examination must be made from the standpoint of the health care professional with the objective of identifying a socially endorsable strategy for interacting with the patient.[8]

The upshot is that clinical moral dilemmas are characteristically problems faced by health professionals about possible interventions in the lives of patients. Given the general role of the ethicist as facilitator of moral inquiry, the clear suggestion is that the primary consulting role should be as advisor to the health professional. These same considerations apply, mutatis mutandis, to situations involving clearly incompetent patients, such as newborn infants. In the latter situations, the health professional is faced with the analogous problem of evaluating the capability of family members or others as proxy decision makers and the implications of this assessment for therapeutic interaction.

Recognition that the ethicist serves primarily as a consultant to the health professional raises the important issue of how the ethicist gains moral authorization to serve in this capacity. The first step in answering this question is to clarify the institutional context in which consultations occur. Normally, they transpire within the confines of an institution of which the ethicist is a salaried employee. Moreover, the ethicist is an administratively authorized resource for use by the primary care provider in enhancing the quality of patient care. (In this respect, the ethicist is functioning in a way similar to the pharmacy or radiologic staff). Finally, being a resource provided by the institution, the ethicist does not receive a separate fee from the patient for consultation services. Although other institutional arrangements may obtain, this is the typical setting for ethics consultations.

Within this framework, two requirements appear sufficient to provide moral authorization for the consulting ethicist: (1) the presumed or actual consent of the patient, and (2) the request of the attending physician.

(1) The physician's own authorization is secured through the patient's acceptance of the former's commitment to serve officiously the goals of the therapeutic relationship. This commitment includes as a standard feature the tacit promise of the physician to place at his disposal institutional resources which will enhance the quality of patient care. Thus, the patient's agreement to enter the therapeutic relationship carries an implied consent to the use of available and useful ancillary services. For example, when the patient enters the hospital we think that there is a tacit agreement that the physician may consult the pharmacist about appropriate drug dosages or selection of optimally effective drugs. The implied consent authorizing consultation with an ethicist can be conceived in a similar fashion.

Naturally, implied consent by the patient can be overridden by the patient's actual refusal to allow the physician to consult the resident ethicist. Moreover, the physician is duty-bound to clear such consultation where it is suspected that there might be such a refusal. It is also the prerogative of the primary physician to seek the patient's actual consent in all cases.

(2) The terms of the physician's original commitment to the patient requires that the physician assess the provisional advisability (subject to the patient's actual or presumed consent) of drawing upon other institutional resources to enhance the quality of patient care. Moreover, as suggested above, the primary role of the ethicist is as a consultant to the physician about the moral dimensions of interaction with the patient. Thus, the request of the physician for a consultation constitutes a second necessary condition for the moral authorization of the consulting ethicist.

Having introduced these general conditions, however, it is important to point out that the way in which the ethicist receives information about the case may alter the conditions required for authorization. In some situations the case may be described to the ethicist without revealing the personal identity of the patient. In this circumstance, requiring the presumed or actual consent of the patient may be too strong a condition. On the other hand, there will be situations in which the ethicist's involvement in the case will include personal interaction with the patient. Obviously, this manner of involvement should require the actual consent of the patient. Finally, there will be consulting situations in which the ethicist does not interact with or observe interactions with the patient, but in which the ethicist has access to information in the patient's medical record. It is this latter type of situation which is most accurately covered by the general position on authorization outlined above.

Acceptance of a consultative role implies that the ethicist accepts the same moral conditions which bring into existence the authorization of the primary care provider. That is, the ethicist must profess or act upon the same bond of loyalty to act on the patient's behalf. In the case of the ethicist, this loyalty involves the specific commitment to direct the process of moral inquiry in a way likely to yield decisions about therapeutic interaction with the patient which would be socially endorsable and effective in operation. But the general duty of the ethicist to serve the patient is precisely similar to that of any other health professionals who apply their special expertise in a consulting patient care role.

Although the involvement of the ethicist is based upon the primary health care provider's commitment to act on behalf of the patient, it does not follow that the health professional has a moral obligation to consult the ethicist whenever a moral problem arises. Rather, the primary consideration is whether the clinician possesses the knowledge of concepts and skills in moral analysis necessary to carry through the process of moral inquiry. The certitude with which he or she is able to draw a conclusion regarding a socially endorsable decision is also an important consideration. In these respects, the situation is quite analogous to the conditions under which a general practitioner might be obligated to consult a specialist. When he or she lacks the necessary skills or is uncertain in clinical judgment regarding a particular aspect of the patient's condition, a consultation is indicated. Thus, Robertson seems quite right in drawing the conclusion that the health professional is sometimes obligated to consult an ethicist.[9] However, there are clear limitations upon this duty, quite similar to the limits upon the moral obligation to request the assistance of other consulting specialists.

While the ethicist serves the health care professional as a consultant and is authorized by the latter's original commitment to the patient, we have yet to specify what services are to be provided in the consulting role. Should ethicists serve only as analysts -- clarifying options, outlining alternative reasons, etc.? Or should they also deliver "correct" conclusions about morally appropriate strategies for therapeutic interaction? Reflection upon the nature of moral inquiry allows us to resolve these issues.

There is little disagreement that the ethicist should at least serve as a problem analyst. The appropriateness of this function is confirmed by considering the ethicist's role as a facilitator of moral inquiry and the various analytic procedures involved. These procedures include identification of problematic

154

values, formulation of problem-solving options, experimental comparison of their operational effectiveness (giving reasons), and investigation of relevant empirical conditions. As facilitator of moral inquiry, the ethicist should identify these various analytic procedures and assist in instituting them in cooperation with the health professionals who are consulted.

But there are serious objections to the claim that the ethicist should provide "right answers" for health professionals. This view derives from an incorrect understanding of the nature of moral inquiry. Moral inquiry is a reflective process that, in part, seeks to formulate plans for therapeutic interaction which in operation will effectively achieve **socially endorsable** outcomes. Morally appropriate behavior cannot be determined apart from the input of various parties to the decision making process regarding the commitments which they would accept upon reflection. Since justified moral commitments are socially produced outcomes, the ethicist cannot claim to know what is morally right in the therapeutic context without participating in this social investigative process. A more pretentious role makes sense only if there are correct moral conclusions which exist independently of human choice and which can only be discovered by the consulting ethicist using special investigative skills.[10]

However, this thesis concerning the social character of moral inquiry does not preclude the permissibility of the ethicist making recommendations for dealing with particular cases. This point is significant since, as Brody points out, "the clinical consultant who advertises in advance that he will not give answers can be guaranteed a great deal of leisure and relatively few consultations."[11] But it is **crucial** that the ethicist and the health care professionals with whom he or she consults clearly understand the status of these recommendations. They are not assertions that such-and-such is the morally correct course of action. They may be claims about the particular problematic values, options, experimental results, or factual data which the ethicist, as one member of the moral community among others, thinks worthy of consideration. Most importantly, though, a recommendation regarding the resolution of a particular problematic case should be a claim about the course of action which the ethicist believes would be effective and endorsed by all members of the moral community who also engage in moral inquiry. This means that such a recommendation cannot be accepted by health professionals who seek consultation unless they also participate in the investigative process. In making a recommendation, the ethicist must underscore the fact that his or her conclusion cannot stand independently of the confirmatory reflection and experience of the health professionals who are consulted. Facilitating this independent investigation is thus a crucial part of the consulting process.[12]

This description of the role of the consulting ethicist allows us to assess the cautionary remarks of Nielsen and Caplan. On one hand, both correctly expose the danger of the idea that ethicists should provide "right answers" for health professionals based upon a knowledge of moral theory. Nielsen points out that this role would require "a systematic knowledge of right and wrong" which current moral theory cannot provide.[13] Moreover, Caplan notes that "Such a view discourages those doing applied ethics from taking seriously what health professionals have to say about moral issues in medicine....(and) discourages close attention to the realities of illness and anxiety for patients and their families."[14] On the other hand, neither Nielsen nor Caplan recognize the legitimate role for the consulting ethicist as a facilitator of the social process of moral reflection and choice. Nielsen fails to see that absence of "a systematic knowledge of right and wrong" does not logically preclude the ethicist from serving as a facilitator of moral inquiry in the manner described above. Similarly, Caplan fails to identify any clear alternative to the "moral engineer" model. The best he can do is to offer advice that "moral engineers" be more conscientious in combining "practical knowledge" and "experience" with their theoretical understanding of moral philosophy.[15]

While the foregoing discussion attempts a positive description of the ethicist's function as consultant, it is equally important to identify other responsibilities which may be mistakenly ascribed to or assumed by ethicists. Brody perceptively notes that these distinctions develop with experience:

> Over time, by observing when the consultation requests... seem appropriate and when they do not, the consultant will devise ways to interact more actively with his primary care colleagues...He will use these opportunities to educate the attending physicians further on what questions his expertise allows him to answer and what questions are really outside his realm...In the process...the consultant may well have been educated by the attending physicians on how he himself ought to define his special area of expertise.[16]

In my own activities as a consultant, several roles have emerged as outside the ethicist's "special area of expertise."

One is the role of moral policeman. On this model, the ethicist's function is to expose activities of health professionals which are clearly immoral. Both health professionals who are not familiar with medical ethics and "activist" or ideologically-oriented ethicists may make this mistake. Societal control of clearly wrong behavior is a task shared by all members of the moral community. By contrast, the specific function of the ethicist relates to medical situations which evoke moral inquiry because the right thing to do is not immediately obvious even to the morally conscientious person. Facilitating moral inquiry and identifying moral improprieties are two quite different undertakings.

A second misconception views the ethicist as a modified social worker. Medical situations exist in which moral goals are clear, but some serious practical obstacle prevents realization of these goals -- for example, when persons are financially unable to purchase air-conditioning units for relief of breathing difficulties.[17] Whereas the latter kind of situation is one in which the problem involves instituting the means to a recognized end, the consulting ethicist's task is to facilitate the investigative process in situations where the problem resolution involves clarification of goals.

A third model inappropriately ascribed to the ethicist is that of secular clergy person. One function of the clerical role is to encourage attitudinal changes which make persons more willing to engage in morally appropriate behavior. The ethicist is sometimes thought to have a similar affective function. By contrast, the role of the ethicist is predominantly intellectual -- fostering the analytic-experimental process most likely to achieve the objective of moral inquiry. Of course, reflective examination is likely to make moral agents more sensitive to the various components of situations which bear upon moral choice. But the attitudinal commitment to do what is morally right is a precondition of the willingness to engage in the process of moral inquiry.

A more subtle mistake is to view the medical ethicist as a patient advocate. On one hand, the ethicist does have a general obligation to the patient to serve the goals of the therapeutic relationship. This involves facilitating moral inquiry that issues in socially endorsable and effective plans for therapeutic interaction with the patient. In this sense, the ethicist certainly is a patient advocate. On the other hand, a patient advocate might be conceived as an agent who defends patients against actions which are clearly violative of their moral or legal rights. Assignment of this function to the ethicist involves the same mistake as the moral policeman model. The special function of the ethicist is not to defend patients against moral wrongdoing, but to facilitate inquiry in situations where the morally correct action is not clear.

Each of these mistaken role assignments results from the failure to distinguish the kind of moral problem with which the consulting ethicist deals from other kinds of situations loosely characterizable as "moral problems." The ethicist addresses situations in which the problem is to settle a conflict of moral values through reflective social choice. By contrast, other kinds of "moral" problems include situations in which (a) some pattern of behavior is morally wrong and needs to be corrected, (b) the actors do not have the attitudinal willingness to engage in morally correct behaviors, or (c) the means for achieving settled moral goals are absent. Failure to distinguish these varieties of moral problems from the type addressed by the consulting ethicist also accounts for several of the "illegitimate roles" described by Thomasma in his essay.[18]

Medical Ethics Pedagogy

While consultation is itself an educational process, the teaching of medical ethics is not restricted to the consultative setting. Development of a systematic approach to medical ethics instruction requires examination of three questions. First, what are the background conditions which form the context of medical ethics teaching? Second, in light of these factors, what should be the primary objectives of medical ethics instruction for health professionals? Finally, what strategies for designing and implementing medical ethics instruction will be most effective in achieving the goals formulated?

Several significant factors provide the background conditions which must be covered in formulating instructional goals. First, the intellectual queries of health professionals regarding moral issues are exceedingly practice-oriented. Health professionals confront recurrent moral decisions in relationships with patients, other health professionals, and society. It is enlightenment in reflecting upon these choices that health professionals seek. Although moral inquiry is initially evoked by situations in which the significance of existing circumstances for present action is unclear, some aspects of moral inquiry and instruction are quite removed from the exigencies of practical decision making -- the subject-matters of general normative theory and metaethics being prime examples. By contrast, instruction in medical ethics must be acutely sensitive to the practical focus of the health professional's daily endeavors.

The proclivity of philosophers to "generalize" rather than "apply" is legend. But the tendency to develop subject-matters relevant to medical practice on their own account is constantly encountered in the medical curriculum -- whether the discipline be anatomy, biochemistry or medical ethics. Thus, Brody notes the tendency of some basic science instructors to induce in medical students an attitude of "progressive incompetence," rather than the capacity to analyze clinical problems in anatomical, biochemical or physiological terms.[19] The same dangers await the medical ethics instructor. But double jeopardy is created by the fact that medical students typically have less acquired interest in humanistic as contrasted with scientific subject-matter.

A second background factor concerns the sophistication and completeness of our moral knowledge. For most situations in which differing values suggest conflicting plans of action, there does not exist socially recognized and settled ways of ordering our moral commitments. An example is the status of the debate concerning medical care for seriously impaired newborns. Moreover, in situations where some moral commitments are settled, there are few well-defined mechanisms for implementing these commitments. For example, although the importance of respect for autonomy in the setting of human research is well-established as a social commitment, mechanisms for assuring effective informed consent have not been well investigated and defined.

A third background factor is the scarcity of available ethics consultants, a point alluded to by Robertson in his essay. There are very few medical universities in which the official duties of the ethics faculty include the provision of consultations. Even fewer consulting ethicists are available in the setting of private medical practice. In addition, as Robertson notes, a recent survey by the President's Commission for the Study of Ethical Problems in Medicine and Biomedical and Behavioral Research indicates that only a very low percentage of hospitals maintain so-called "ethics committees" which might serve in a consultative role.[20] Assuming no forseeable change in this situation, health professionals will usually need to address moral issues in consultation only with colleagues.

These three factors regarding professional practice -- the press of practical decision making, the absence of social recipes for resolving moral issues, and the scarcity of ethics consultants -- suggest that the focus of medical ethics teaching should be development of the independent capacity of health professionals to apply the method of moral inquiry in resolving case-oriented problems in health care practice. Development of fluency in using the method of moral inquiry requires that at least five elements comprise medical ethics instruction. First, students must be introduced to the variety of moral dilemmas which arise in clinical practice. Familiarity with this typology of issues helps to effectively assure that significant moral dilemmas will not be overlooked or improperly conceptualized. Second, they must clearly understand the objectives of moral inquiry -- its status as a process of social decision making which seeks to formulate effective and publicly endorsable policies for resolving morally problematic situations. Otherwise, moral reflection may be improperly identified with such things as "consulting conscience," applying personal religious beliefs, or recalling mores learned in the course of health professional training. Third, health professionals must become familiar with the analytic steps of moral inquiry and gain skill in applying these procedures in the decision making process regarding particular problematic situations.

A fourth goal is the introduction of moral principles and conceptual distinctions which facilitate the process of moral inquiry. On one hand, the "middle level" moral principles mentioned earlier -- such as respect for autonomy, concern for the well-being of particular persons, justice or fairness, promotion of the general well-being of society, promisekeeping, etc. -- direct attention to the features of the consequences of alternative plans of action which must be considered in deliberative and experimental comparison leading to social choices. On the other hand, various conceptual distinctions provide tools for clarifying morally relevant differences among situations in which a particular issue arises. For example, the distinction between competent and incompetent decision making may provide a morally useful strategy for distinguishing different circumstances in which a policy is sought regarding refusal of treatment. Taken together, principles and conceptual distinctions represent the intellectual fund of moral experience and constitute methodological tools which may be useful in resolving present moral problems.

A final goal is the introduction of health professionals to social science data which bear upon the analysis and resolution of clinical moral dilemmas. While Graber succinctly summarizes the other objectives of medical ethics instruction, he fails to consider the importance of this additional goal.[21] Similarly, although Reynolds, Eaddy, and Swander rightly emphasize the importance of clinical experience in the development of discerning moral judgment, they fail to note that systematic knowledge of the psychosocial aspects of clinical interaction enhances the quality of moral reflection.[22] There is a growing body of knowledge in anthropology, psychiatry, social psychology and sociology directly relevant to moral issues in the therapeutic relationship. Since fact-finding is an essential component of moral reflection, introduction of this material is also an important instructional goal.

Formulation of strategies for implementing medical ethics instruction in the professional curriculum is as crucially important as the clarification of instructional objectives. Discussion of teaching strategies will focus upon both the choice of appropriate curriculum settings and the ways in which general instructional goals should be implemented within these settings. Brevity requires that these matters be examined only in the context of the medical school curriculum. However, the general approach is applicable with appropriate modifications in the training of other health professionals.

Our experience at The University of Tennessee Center for the Health Sciences has suggested the importance of one fundamental strategy: medical ethics instruction, where possible, should be integrated into existing curriculum structures of the medical school. There are several reasons supporting this approach. First, creation of new curriculum devices (such as graduate-style seminars once every two weeks) may meet more administrative resistance than the integration of medical ethics teaching into established curriculum structures. Second, use of recognized medical teaching modalities is likely to lead to more ready acceptance by students of medical ethics instruction than the use of formats foreign to the usual pattern of medical education. Third, medical ethics instruction within established curriculum structures lends itself to participation by students and faculty whose pattern of attendance at teaching functions is circumscribed within the usual departmental schedules. Finally, implementation in existing curriculum structures reinforces the conception among students that medical ethics teaching is as integral to medical education as discussions of diagnosis, prognosis, and treatment of disease states.

Illustration of these points may be provided by reference to the case conference format in medical education. A standard feature of the medical curriculum is the conference which focuses upon some aspect of a particular case history, as is often done in the grand rounds setting. The strategy outlined above suggests that medical ethics instruction should be inserted into grand rounds sessions which occur as part of the regular conference schedule of clinical departments. For example, Ethics Grand Rounds at the Center for the Health Sciences occurs as part of the grand rounds schedule in five core clinical departments. For the reasons discussed above, our observations indicate that this approach is more effective than the previous strategy of conducting Ethics Grand Rounds as an independent function of the Program on Human Values and Ethics, not coordinated with the conference schedule of core departments.

If the fundamental strategy is accepted, then the medical ethics curriculum must be developed by patterning its settings and implementation of instructional goals upon the general structure of medical education. The standard undergraduate medical curriculum is divided between basic science and clinical components. The function of the basic science curriculum is to provide the student with the ability to analyze clinical problems using the conceptual resources of various "background" disciplines, such as anatomy, physiology and biochemistry. The teaching format used in the basic science years consists predominantly of lectures and laboratories.

In analogous fashion, this portion of the curriculum might include a section on ethics devoted to the provision of background knowledge which will prepare the student to analyze clinical care decisions from a moral standpoint. With regard to the general goals of medical ethics instruction, this background must include an understanding of what moral inquiry is and a familiarity with its constitutive analytic procedures. It might also introduce the main conceptions which are useful in analyzing all clinical moral problems, particularly the "middle-level" moral principles. Finally, it must provide an overview of the main types of moral issues which arise in relations with patients, fellow professionals and society -- e.g., conflicts between respect for patients' wishes and concern for their well-being, or between pursuit of the well-being of society and concern for the interests of particular patients.

This general introduction to clinical ethics can be accomplished using the lecture format of basic science education. The format is, however, profitably supplemented by case discussion sessions which illustrate the types of issues encountered and the use of moral inquiry as a method of social decision making. Use of this latter supplement functions pedagogically in a role similar to the basic science laboratory.

In contrast to the basic science curriculum, virtually all medical education in the clinical years is accomplished in individual specialties or departments. The function of this portion of the curriculum is to introduce principles of clinical care -- its diagnostic and therapeutic components -- within the context of particular specialties such as internal medicine, surgery, obstetrics and gynecology, pediatrics and psychiatry. Within each specialty, there are a number of standard teaching modalities: lectures, case conferences, teaching rounds, seminars, and participation in patient care.

Integration of medical ethics instruction into this structure of specialty-oriented clinical education requires that its general goals be implemented while focusing upon ethical issues arising in the respective core specialities (e.g., treatment for defective newborns in pediatrics, determinations of competence in psychiatry). Within the framework of this restricted focus, implementation of general instructional goals will have several components. One is the provision of a typology of major issues arising within the particular clinical specialty, which will facilitate the ability of students to identify common moral problems. Another component is the introduction of conceptual distinctions which are especially useful in addressing these issues. Within the psychiatric setting, for instance, examination of the conceptual aspects of competence would obviously be appropriate. A third feature is the presentation of factual data relative to the resolution of clinical care issues. In the pediatric setting, information on quality of life outcomes for seriously ill neonates would be directly relevant to discussion of decisions to terminate treatment. The most important component, however, may be enhancement of the ability of students to utilize the analytic procedures of moral inquiry in examining patient care decisions. Graber's emphasis upon this latter point is well-taken.[23]

Standard teaching modalities available in the clinical curriculum can be selectively utilized in achieving different goals. For example, clerkship lectures are an appropriate setting for introducing the typology of issues, relevant conceptual distinctions, and significant factual data. On the other hand, clinical case conferences and teaching rounds are useful teaching contexts within which the procedures of moral inquiry can be illustrated and practiced. When available, seminars provide for more in-depth analysis of particular issues and extended examination of representative case histories.

Implementation of medical ethics instruction in the clinical curriculum requires that the ethicist attain what might be called "clinical credibility." Clinical credibility involves the judgement of colleagues within a particular medical specialty that the ethicist has a legitimate contribution to make in the clinical education of students. Achievement of clinical credibility involves a number of factors. One requirement is that the ethicist secure sufficient knowledge of the clinical specialty to clearly understand the clinical dimensions of common moral issues and to fluently discuss these issues with clinical colleagues and students. A second factor is that the ethicist gain "recognition" as a colleague through regular attendance at various teaching functions within the department. Another prerequisite is that the ethicist attain considerable facility in communicating the role of moral inquiry and introducing its analytic procedures and conceptual tools within the constraints of available teaching modalities.

Gaining clinical credibility within a particular core medical specialty requires substantial commitment of time and learning effort on the part of the ethicist. As a result, the clinical teaching involvement of particular ethics faculty members must be restricted in focus to a single clinical specialty or closely related medical specialties. At The University of Tennessee Center for the Health Sciences, this recognition has resulted in the develoment of a consultative-liaison model for the involvement of medical ethics faculty in the clinical medical curriculum. According to this model, each ethics faculty member attends teaching rounds, participates in ethics case conferences, presents clerkship lectures, etc. within the particular specialty. Our initial assessment of this model for involvement suggests that it is an effective mechanism for achieving clinical credibility of the ethicist and for implementing a clinical medical ethics curriculum patterned upon the general structure of clinical medical education.

Medical Ethics Investigation

Moral dilemmas in health care practice arise when distinct values suggest conflicting courses of action and a lack of consensus exists concerning the pattern of social interaction to be instituted. The goal of moral inquiry is to identify plans of action which are socially endorsable because they will effectively secure the outcomes which members of the moral community cherish upon reflection. The method of investigation optimal in achieving this goal is not determinable in an a priori fashion. Rather, it must be identified by comparative evaluation of alternative methods with respect to their effectiveness in achieving the goal of moral inquiry. This is true in any field of investigation. The experimental procedures of medical science, such as its recently expanded biostatistical component, have not descended from the a priori blue. Preferred methods have been identified by their ability to yield experimental results which achieve the goal of such inquiry -- the correlation of biophysical changes. Thus, the fundamental question is: what method of moral inquiry will be most productive in yielding norms that are effective in operation and evocative of a genuinely shared social commitment? Three options will be examined: the deductive model of recent moral philosophy, the method of classical casuistry, and the experimental approach outlined earlier in this paper.

Nielsen carefully reviews the frustrated efforts of recent moral theory to construct "a systematic knowledge of right and wrong" applicable to the resolution of practical moral dilemmas.[24] His analysis raises two questions for the comparative evaluation of methods: First, are there shortcomings in the methodology of recent moral philosophy which might account for this failure? Second, does the failure to develop such systematic knowledge mean, as Nielsen suggests, that we cannot make headway in resolving moral issues in clinical medicine?

The method of recent moral theory involves several components. First, it assumes that resolution of practical moral dilemmas requires prior agreement regarding fundamental moral principles. Second, concrete moral issues are to be settled by logically deducing solutions from a statement of the fundamental principle(s) and a statement of the relevant facts of the situation(s) under examination. Third, fundamental principles are to be selected by persons making choices under constraints constitutive of "the moral point of view." The method is pseudo-mathematical, with the axioms of the system being chosen under certain restrictive conditions rather than arbitrarily.[25]

The method has two critical defects which, I believe, account for its relative infertility in addressing bioethical dilemmas. First, the facts about dilemmatic situations do not enter into the development of principles, but are relevant in a significant way only in their **application** to problems of medical practice. Of course, characterization of the moral point of view usually includes the proviso that choices be made in light of relevant factual knowledge. But in the context of choices of fundamental principles, this knowledge includes only the barest generalities about human nature and social behavior. It does not include attention to the empirical dimensions of the problematic situations which give rise to moral inquiry.

With empirical development, test and revision of moral norms ruled out, there is limited recourse in resolving disputes which arise regarding the appropriate content of fundamental norms. On one hand, the inadequacy of opposing views can only be shown by establishing that they have fallen prey to some logical inconsistency within the moral point of view. On the other hand, the only claim that can be made in support of a favored principle is to show that it is consistent with other principles chosen. The possibility of experimental investigation of alternative norms in their operational impact upon valued outcomes in actual situations is replaced by interminable analytic debates regarding the possible meanings and logical implications of moral principles which are proposed. The result is a methodological dilemma: the appeal to mere logical consistency of choices within the moral point of view is found inadequate in identifying norms which evoke a genuinely shared social commitment, while the employment of further investigative procedures which may yield a social consensus is foreclosed by the **a priori** limitations of the accepted method.

The second fundamental defect of the investigative method of recent moral theory relates to the deductive process by which fundamental norms are "applied" to practical moral dilemmas. By their very nature, basic moral principles portray generalized goals or modes of social interaction to which common allegiance is recommended. As a result, they cannot carry as part of their very meaning an implied selection of the plans or outcomes to be cherished in the very specific circumstances which characterize concrete moral dilemmas. For example, suppose it is granted that the principle of beneficence is the relevant norm in settling the issue of how to provide further medical care to an incompetent patient. In promoting the patient's well-being, how is prolongation of life to be balanced against maintenance of its quality? With respect to its quality, how shall various factors such as ambulation, communicative capacity and freedom from pain be prioritized? The principle itself does not carry the solution to these questions. As a result, "application" of the principle really involves a development of its content. Logically speaking, this develoment involves setting priorities among possible valued outcomes and related plans.

This feature of the deductive method suggests the second reason for its failure to be productive in resolving practical moral issues. Even where basic principles are points of common agreement, conflicts arise regarding their interpretation in concrete situations. Proponents of one way of setting priorities among valued outcomes or plans of action produce one specification of the principle, while those favoring another pattern of priorities provide an alternative "deduction." In reality, both parties are reading the result of a favored priority-seeking back into the meaning of the fundamental principle. But when either side then appeals to the principle as the justificatory basis for adopting a particular plan of action, the logical circle is complete. Since the rules of the deductive method make appeal to fundamental principles the means for resolving conflicts, no further resolutory strategy is available for breaking through the separate logical circles to achieve a shared commitment.

In light of these defects of the deductive model, the second issue raised by Nielsen's discussion becomes crucial. Is he right to insist that we cannot make headway in resolving moral issues in clinical medicine without first attaining a "systematic knowledge of right and wrong"? I suggest that the experimental method constitutes an alternative approach which provides more effective procedural resources for achieving the goal of moral inquiry. Moreover, it does not necessitate prior establishment of the systematic knowledge of which Nielsen speaks.

Different types of moral issues arise under very specific kinds of empirical conditions, while alternative approaches to their resolution create distinctive empirical consequences. How are resolutions to be achieved which realize and reflect the considered valuings of all persons? The experimental method involves several key steps. First, claims about what morally ought to be done are to be treated as **hypotheses** regarding the forms of social interaction which will be effective in realizing outcomes reflectively valued by persons in the circumstances which create the moral problem. Second, identification of a socially endorsable plan of action is to proceed by comparative evaluation of alternative plans in their capacity to interact with existing empirical conditions to achieve these valued outcomes. Third, the projected outcomes of alternative plans are to be compared with their actual outcomes in concrete operation. The revision of cherished outcomes and/or hypotheses (plans) proceeds until an effective and socially endorsable plan can be achieved.

This experimental approach takes us beyond choice of principles by mere logical consistency within the moral point of view,

and provides the opportunity for a consenses regarding bioethical
norms to emerge from hypothesis-directed development of correlations between policy options and their consequences for outcomes
valued by members of the moral community. Moreover, while the
deductive method only allows priorities in concrete situations to
be surreptitiously read back into the meaning of the principles
from which they are supposedly "deduced," the experimental
approach requires that these priorities be formulated as hypotheses and investigated in their actual empirical outcome.

Finally, the experimental method does not require that we
first attain a "systematic knowledge of right and wrong" before
resolutions to biomedical moral dilemmas can be developed.
Rather, tentative solutions to each type of moral dilemma must
first be developed through hypothesis-directed investigation of
the circumstances in which it arises. These solutions are plans
of action expected to realize the outcomes which members of the
moral community reflectively cherish in these situations.
Through comparison of tentative solutions to different dilemmas,
recurrent features of justified plans of action and outcomes get
identified. These generalized notions are formulated as moral
principles. They are then available as tools of analysis in
examining new moral problems or in revising tentative solutions
to current dilemmas. In this sense general knowledge about right
and wrong can be developed to provide an important resource in
addressing biomedical moral issues. But this is hardly the
finished system of moral principles which Nielsen would maintain
must be constructed before we can begin to resolve moral
dilemmas in medical practice.

One objection to the experimental approach might insist that
scientific methodology is only useful in developing knowledge
about "what is the case," whereas bioethics is concerned with
"what we morally ought to do." The reply involves two points.
First, it is admitted that bioethical inquiry concerns commitments to bring certain states of affairs into existence, whereas
scientific research deals merely with the correlation of changes
which actually do ensue when empirical conditions are transformed
via experimentation. But plans of action and valued outcomes
gain "obligatory status" insofar as they will be effective in
operation and evocative of a shared social commitment. Thus, the
crucial question involves how such commitments are to be
developed.

Second, the relevance of the experimental method to their
development is suggested by the fact that valued plans and outcomes are as much observable phenomena as biophysical changes.
Having a particular moral commitment involves striving to
achieve, avoid, maintain or eliminate certain states of affairs.
Moreover, these states of affairs will affect the realization of
other values in interaction with the empirical factors which

constitute the conditions and consequences of these moral commitments. As a result, the formation of shared social commitments can be intellectually controlled by comparative examination of alternative plans of action in their impact upon valued outcomes under the conditions which characterize morally problematic situations. In particular, formulation of possible plans of action as hypotheses can direct action and observation until a plan of action is found which effectively achieves an integrated set of valued outcomes endorsed by members of the moral community.

Thus, the experimental approach involves no denial of the "is-ought" distinction. Rather, it insists that moral commitments having the status of mere occurrences are distinguished from those which have normative status because the latter have been formed according to whatever method optimally yields norms satisfying the goal of moral inquiry. The foregoing argument has suggested the special advantages of the experimental method **vis a vis** the deductive model in identifying such norms.

In sharp contrast to Nielsen's unquestioning allegiance to the investigative methodology of recent moral theory, Jonsen undertakes a novel effort to develop the relevance of classical casuistry to moral problems in medicine.[26] There are several respects in which the casuistical method exhibits clear advantages over the investigative approach of recent moral theory. First, it has a more satisfactory understanding of the goal of moral inquiry. Comparing the casuistical approach to the deductive model, Jonsen writes:

> ...its aim was not to lead the mind, through ineluctable steps of formal argument, to a compelling truth, but to reveal, by juxtaposition of maxims and circumstances, an option that could reasonably be entertained...Its aim is persuasion: not to be understood as swaying gullible minds by specious reasons, but leading reflective minds to reasonable opinions about those things, which by their nature cannot be demonstrated formally... Classical casuistry was eminently practical. Its aim was not only to understand a moral problem but to resolve it.[27]

Implicit in these comments is the suggestion that a moral problem presents a situation in which there is a lack of consensus regarding the pattern of social interaction to be instituted. Moreover, in describing casuistry as "eminently practical," there is recognition that the goal of moral inquiry is to achieve reflective identification of shared norms which allows an integrated pattern of social interaction to go forward.

Second, casuistry clearly recognizes that achieving the goal of moral inquiry requires painstaking analysis of concrete moral situations. The reflective movement from paradigms to analogies via the examination of possible circumstances allows for examination of the differential import of varied conditions and consequences. This stands in sharp contrast to the deductive model, where particular circumstances play a substantial role only in the application of "systematic knowledge of right and wrong" to specific moral problems. As already suggested, it is more likely that plans which evoke a genuinely shared social commitment can be engendered by a method which starts with careful analysis of morally problematic situations than with one that proceeds from fundamental principles.

Finally, the casuistical approach has a more satisfactory understanding of the role of maxims (principles) in moral inquiry than the deductive method of recent moral theory. In casuistry, maxims are not used as preselected axioms from which the resolutions to particular moral problems are "deduced." Thus, Jonsen writes that:

> ...casuists never attempt to systematize
> maxims: They do not use them as axioms to
> construct an argument; they do not marshal
> them into lexical orderings; they do not even
> worry much about "justifying" them. They
> simply invoke them, much as ordinary folk do
> in arguing moral matters.[28]

In effect, maxims serve the same function as principles in the experimental approach. They are tools of analysis, which provide reflective persons with categories in terms of which the "circumstances" characterizing particular situations are to be considered in arriving at acceptable moral solutions. Thus, casuistry avoids the problems of settling upon fundamental principles in abstraction from concrete circumstances, and of establishing non-circular "deductions" from such principles. These latter problems undermine the usefulness of the deductive model in achieving the goal of moral inquiry.

Nevertheless, there are serious defects in the casuistical approach which, I believe, are properly remedied by use of the experimental method. First, the goal of moral inquiry includes the identification of plans of action which not only evoke a shared social commitment, but which are also **effective** in actually achieving valued outcomes under the conditions which characterize morally problematic situations. As described by Jonsen, the casuistical method relies upon thoughtful deliberation concerning paradigms, analogies and circumstances in examining the operation of various courses of action in the situations which create a moral dilemma. Although thoughtful deliberation may sometimes be all that the exigencies of decision making allow, such "imaginative rehearsal" involves little more than spelling out the lessons of past experience for the moral problem currently under investigation.[29] This imaginative deliberation cannot replace the usefulness of prospective evaluation of policy options. Comparative prospective examination of alternative plans in their concrete effectiveness can be optimized only if they are treated as hypotheses which direct implementation and observation of their actual outcomes **vis a vis** alternative plans. Thus, the casuistical approach fails to avail itself of the opportunity to employ experimental procedures in developing and revising plans and valued outcomes so as to achieve effective patterns of social interaction.

A second problem inherent in the casuistical approach is closely related. Jonsen notes that casuistry involves determining which maxims "fit" particular circumstances. However, no clear position is articulated regarding the conditions under which a solution "fits" the morally dilemmatic situations to which it is applied. Without a clear conception of the "fittingness" of a solution, the procedures of the casuistical approach cannot guide us in achieving solutions to moral dilemmas.

This conceptual dilemma regarding the "fittingness" of plans can be addressed in two steps. First, it requires a clear conception of the goal of moral inquiry. This goal is to develop plans for resolving morally problematic situations which engender a social consensus because they are effective in achieving outcomes valued by members of the moral community. A solution "fits" morally problematic circumstances if it has these properties of effectiveness and shared commitment. Presumably, the casuistical method could accept this much by way of clarification of the notion of "fittingness."

Second, clarification of the concept of "fittingness" also requires a specification of the investigative procedures which will be most useful in determining whether a **particular** plan of action "fits" the moral dilemma to which it is applied. Much of the previous argument has been devoted to outlining the advantages of hypothesis-directed experimentation, observation, and subsequent revision of plans in arriving at solutions to moral problems in medicine which satisfy the goal of moral inquiry. It is not clear what resources are available on the casuistical approach for bringing maxims and circumstances into appropriate juxtaposition, save the process of thoughtful deliberation which attempts to compare and distinguish conceivable circumstances. By contrast, operational examination of alternative plans of actions provides a mechanism for "mapping" possible solutions onto morally problematic situations to determine their "fit."

A final problem concerns the status of "maxims" in the investigative process. The crucial role of maxims in the casuistical approach is clear: solutions are found by fitting maxims to circumstances. These maxims are, in Jonsen's words, "the common coin of moral discourse," ranging from "platitudes" to "the solid commonplaces of morality."[30] But insofar as they are common stock, they represent conventional moral wisdom. Thus, a serious criticism is that casuistry embodies a deep moral conservatism that may obstruct the development of creative solutions to moral dilemmas.

In evaluating this criticism, it is important to recognize that the use of moral principles as tools for analyzing morally problematic situations lends itself, by their very nature, to a certain degree of moral conservatism. If my previous analysis is correct, moral principles summarize general features of plans or valued outcomes which have been found profitable in resolving moral dilemmas in past situations. Thus in directing analysis of policy options and outcomes in present circumstances, moral principles tend to set moral thinking in the direction of previous solutions. But the more important issue is whether or not the casuistical approach includes counterbalancing factors which check the conservative tendencies involved in using moral principles. Unfortunately, Jonsen's description of the method does not provide evidence that it has such neutralizing features.

By contrast, the experimental approach offers an interpretation of the status of moral principles which establishes the nature of both their use and limitation in moral investigation. On one hand, they provide helpful categories, drawn from past moral experience, for analyzing present policy options and valued outcomes. This constitutes their use. On the other hand, they have only tentative application to new moral problems. Their present relevance depends upon their ability to provide analytic guidance leading to policies which are effective in operation and evocative of a social consensus. Insofar as they fail to provide such guidance, they must be revised or dropped. This means that, on the experimental approach, moral principles are subject to the same test of valid use as other conceptual apparatuses of moral investigation -- whether or not they serve as effective means in achieving the goal of moral inquiry. Thus, the experimental approach allows us to draw upon the wisdom of past moral experience as summarized in moral principles, without being trapped by the conventional tendencies which they embody.

The assessment of alternative methods of moral investigation has proceeded by analyzing their comparative effectiveness in achieving the goal of moral inquiry. On one hand, the method of recent moral theory has been found wanting in virtue of its a priori limitations. Selection of fundamental principles in abstraction from concrete moral conditions and difficulties in "applying" these vague generalizations to particular situations render the approach unproductive in identifying effective and socially shared norms. On the other hand, the method of casuistry recognizes the importance of careful analysis of the conditions which characterize morally problematic situations. But it fails to develop a clear understanding of how moral conceptions are to be mapped onto the problematic situations they are intended to resolve. By contrast to these methodological approaches, the experimental method recognizes the conjugate and interdependent role of moral conceptions and empirical conditions in developing solutions to moral problems in medicine. The link between conceptions and circumstances in achieving the goal of moral inquiry is provided by the experimental investigation of alternative plans for resolving these dilemmas.

Adoption of the experimental approach in medical ethics inquiry would necessitate drastic changes in the way such investigation is typically conducted. Plans of action produce valued or disvalued outcomes only in interaction with existing empirical conditions. Consequently, both plans and cherished outcomes can only be selected through careful analysis of these interacting conditions. In the clinical setting, these factors include psychological, sociological and medical circumstances. Despite this fact, it is vanishingly rare to find analyses of moral issues in medicine which build upon painstaking examination of operative empirical factors. Rectification of this situation can only proceed by systematic incorporation of the results of social and medical science investigations into the discussion of clinical moral issues.

Thus, medical ethics inquiry must become an essentially interdisciplinary undertaking. Clinical psychology, sociology, anthropology, and medicine all have contributions to make to the resolution of clinical moral issues. This means not only that ethicists must incorporate the results of investigations in these various disciplines into their analyses of clinical moral dilemmas. More importantly, it implies that problems and methods of investigation developed in these various fields must be formulated in a way that permits data to be accumulated which contributes directly to the resolution of moral issues.

Summary

The foregoing discussion has analyzed the consultative, pedagogical, and investigative methods of medical ethics in the clinical setting. A crucial assumption is that in each mode of activity the medical ethicist functions as a facilitator of the reflective social decision making process constituting moral inquiry. Thus, analysis of the consultative, pedagogical and investigative roles has proceeded by attempting to identify the methods peculiar to each mode of activity which will be the most effective means for achieving the goal of moral inquiry. However much the findings of other investigators may differ regarding these same questions, the touchstone of evaluation must be the comparative capacity of the alternative methods espoused to achieve this goal.

FOOTNOTES

[1]McElhinney and Pellegrino, eds., **HUMAN VALUES TEACHING PROGRAMS FOR HEALTH PROFESSIONALS** (Ardmore, Penn.: Whitmore, 1981).

[2]I would suggest that this same property also describes moral inquiry which occurs within the framework of an accepted theological perspective. A particular religious perspective is constituted by a set of general values or norms which must be applied to or interpreted within the circumstances characterizing concrete moral dilemmas. But "application" actually involves the development of the content of these norms through a process of choice or priority-setting. This point is discussed in more detail in my critique of the deductive model of moral inquiry. See pp. 162-166.

[3]The fine work of the National Commission for the Protection of Human Subjects of Biomedical and Behavioral Research provides an excellent illustration of this aspect of moral inquiry.

[4]John Dewey, **THEORY OF THE MORAL LIFE** (New York: Holt, Rinehart and Winston, 1960), p. 135.

[5]Of course, Veatch would also maintain that the physician has a moral right not to perform services which violate his or her own moral beliefs. However, assuming that the physician's moral commitments are not at stake in the context of a particular moral dilemma, the physician should provide technically competent services under the conditions specified by the patient.

[6]Veatch, "Does a Clinical Role for Medical Ethics Violate or Enhance Therapeutic Relationships?," this volume, p. 60.

[7]Ackerman, "Autonomy and the Constraints of Illness: Why Doctors Should Intervene," **HASTINGS CENTER REPORT** 12 (August, 1982), pp. 14-17; and "Medical Ethics and the Two Dogmas of Liberalism," **THEORETICAL MEDICINE**, 5/1 (February 1984), pp. 69-81.

[8]Insofar as illness typically involves cognitive, affective and social constraints upon autonomous behavior, the health professional must assess in **every** case whether the best way to respect the patient's autonomy is to accept the latter's choice at face value. Even when this conclusion is drawn, the health professional has made a moral decision about interaction with the patient. Moreover, in some cases the correct conclusion will be that some constraint -- such as anxiety, denial, or submission to authority -- impairs the patient's decision making capacity. In this situation formulation of special interactive strategies will be necessary to enhance the patient's autonomy.

Thus, moral decision making by the health professional, **pace** Veatch, is an inescapable element of the therapeutic relationship.

[9]John Robertson, "Clinical Medical Ethics and the Law: Rights and Duties in Ethics Consultations," this volume, pp. 67-80.

[10]One important misunderstanding of this position must be avoided. It is not being suggested that we must canvass the entire moral community before we can identify morally appropriate plans for therapeutic interaction in a particular case. In its fullest sense, this is never possible. Thus, I noted earlier that we seek decisions in moral inquiry which formulate socially endorsable plans of action -- plans that would be upheld by the wider moral community, even if this broader endorsement cannot now be sought. Rather, I am suggesting only that the ethicist cannot claim to identify correct resolutions to clinical moral dilemmas apart from the contribution of other persons who also willingly engage in the analytic-experimental process of moral investigation.

[11]Howard Brody, "Teaching Clinical Ethics: Models for Consideration," this volume, p. 38.

[12]Relevant to this point is an interesting consulting technique described by a participant in my working group at the conference. Dr. Haavi Morreim, University of Virginia Medical Center, provides short "position papers" for health professionals with whom she consults. The function of these papers is to spell out available options and their value implications, so that the parties consulted will be obliged to work through the reflective process of moral inquiry when reviewing the report. As a further incentive to participation by the consulted health professional in the reflective process, she declines to offer a recommendation. The analysis just presented suggests that the need to encourage participation in the reflective process is essential in achieving the goal of moral inquiry and is not merely a Socratic scruple. But I would not consider it necessary (or even desirable) to forego the making of a recommendation, **provided that** the status of the recommendation is properly understood.

[13]Kai Nielsen, "On Being Skeptical About Applied Ethics," this volume, pp. 93-113.

[14]Arthur Caplan, "Can Applied Ethics Be Effective in Health Care and Should It Strive To Be?," this volume, p. 140.

[15]Ibid., p. 138.

[16]Brody, op. cit., p. 39.

[17]Of course, the case described also raises moral issues of the primary sort having to do with the distribution of health care resources.

[18]David Thomasma, "Legitimate and Illegitimate Roles for the Medical Ethicist," this volume, pp. 81-92.

[19]Brody, op. cit.

[20]Robertson, op. cit., p. 70.

[21]Glenn Graber, "Teaching Medical Ethics in the Clinical Setting: Objectives, Strategies, Qualifications," this volume, pp. 1-30.

[22]Charles Reynolds, John Eaddy and Karen Swander, "On Bridging the Theory/Practice Gap in Training Medical Ethicists," this volume, pp. 43-56. Although Reynolds, Eaddy and Swander insist that medical ethicists should receive sociology instruction to develop skills of clinical observation (p. 52), they do not consider the similar importance of the systematic knowledge base available in the social sciences.

[23]Graber, op. cit., pp. 6, 15-16.

[24]Nielsen, "On Being Skeptical About Applied Ethics," this volume, pp. 93-113.

[25]Since John Rawls' method of "reflective equilibrium" has achieved considerable popularity as an approach to the analysis of moral issues, it is useful to state its relationship to what I call the "deductive model." My contention is that, with respect to the resolution of moral problems (as I have defined them), Rawls' approach is a species of the deductive approach. Rawls' fundamental goal is to formulate a theory "...describing our sense of justice" [A THEORY OF JUSTICE (Cambridge: Harvard University Press, 1971), p. 46]. The goal is to be accomplished by developing a coherent body of propositions of four types: conditions to be set upon the choice of fundamental principles (the moral point of view); the fundamental principles themselves; considered judgments in reflective equilibrium; and general factual considerations which must be known to determine how persons would choose within the moral point of view.

Development of the general theory in relatively complete form must occur before embarking upon the effort to resolve morally problematic situations. This point is suggested by the nature of considered judgments. Considered judgments are moral claims which, among other things, we would make without ambivalence or hesitation (A THEORY OF JUSTICE, p. 47). This means that, by definition, they are not moral claims developed within the context of morally problematic situations, where a social consensus is lacking and what we ought to do is uncertain. Since considered judgments are the only "concrete" element used in theory formation, it is clear that this process occurs apart from the context of problematic situations.

Finally, it is then necessary to apply the developed theory to the resolution of morally problematic situations in medical practice. I assume Rawls would require that this be done by deductive application of the general theory, since he believes that the ideal form of the general theory itself would be a set of propositions related in strictly deductive fashion (A THEORY OF JUSTICE, p. 121). Thus, it is most accurate to interpret Rawls' "decision procedure" for ethics as an analysis of how fundamental principles are to be chosen, while the resolution of practical moral dilemmas is to proceed by a deductive application of principles characteristic of all versions of the deductive model.

For Rawls' view regarding moral justification, see A THEORY OF JUSTICE, especially sections 9, 20 and 87.

[26]Albert Jonsen, "On Being a Casuist," this volume, pp. 115–128.

[27]Ibid., pp. 121.

[28]Ibid., p. 120.

[29]Dewey, loc. cit.

[30]Jonsen, op. cit., p. 121.

Notes on Contributors

Terrence F. Ackerman, Ph.D., is Chairman of the Department on Human Values and Ethics, University of Tennessee, Memphis.

Howard Brody, M.D., Ph.D., is an Assistant Professor in the Department of Family Practice and Coordinator, Medical Humanities Program, Michigan State University, East Lansing, Michigan.

Arthur Caplan, Ph.D., is Associate Director, The Hastings Center, Hasting-on-Hudson, New York, and Associate for Social Medicine, Columbia University College of Physicians and Surgeons, New York.

John Eaddy, M.C., is Associate Professor and Deputy Chairman in the Department of Family Practice, University of Tennessee Memorial Research Center and Hospital, and Adjunct Professor of Philosophy at the University of Tennessee-Knoxville, Knoxville, Tennessee.

Glenn Graber, Ph.D., is Professor of Philosophy and Associate Head, Department of Philosophy, University of Tennessee-Knoxville; Clinical Associate in Medical Ethics, University of Tennessee Memorial Research Center and Hospital, Knoxville; and Director of the University Studies Program, UTK.

Albert Jonsen, Ph.D., is Professor of Ethics in Medicine and Chief, Division of Medical Ethics, The School of Medicine, University of California-San Francisco.

Kai Nielsen, Ph.D., is Professor of Philosophy, Department of Philosophy, University of Calgary, Calgary, Alberta, Canada.

Charles Reynolds, Ph.D., is Professor and Chairman, Department of Religious Studies, University of Tennessee-Knoxville, Knoxville, Tennessee.

John Robertson, J.D., is Professor of Law, University of Texas School of Law, Austin, Texas.

Karen Swander, Ph.D. is a counseling psychologist with the student counseling services center and Associate Professor of Educational and Counseling Psychology at the University of Tennessee, Knoxville. She is a diplomat in Counseling Psychology of the American Board of Professional Psychology.

David Thomasma, Ph.D., is Director, Medical Humanities Program, Loyola University Stritch School of Medicine, Chicago, Illinois.

Robert Veatch, Ph.D., is Professor of Medical Ethics, The Kennedy Institute of Ethics, Georgetown University, Washington, D.C.